YOUR SKIN AND HAIR

Earle W. Brauer, M.D.

YOUR SKIN AND HAIR

A BASIC GUIDE TO CARE AND BEAUTY

The Macmillan Company, New York, New York

Collier-Macmillan Ltd., London

Library of Congress Catalog Card Number: 68–28892

Third Printing 1971

The Macmillan Company
866 Third Avenue, New York, N.Y. 10022
Collier-Macmillan Canada Ltd., Toronto, Ontario

PRINTED IN THE UNITED STATES OF AMERICA

FOREWORD

This book is the product of an unusual union of two careers. After twenty years in medicine, the more recent fifteen of which were devoted entirely to the practice and teaching of dermatology, I became, in 1962, first consulting dermatologist and then the medical director of the world's leading cosmetic company. My perspective on the subject of skin care and skin adornment is for these reasons special and unique.

Books about the skin and its hygiene written for laymen by doctors have usually emphasized skin disorders. If the subject of cosmetics was mentioned at all, it was probably in reference to the hiding of birthmarks or the occasional allergy a few persons have exhibited to certain products. On the other hand, fashion magazines and the women's pages of newspapers regularly describe current trends in the use of cosmetics, along with a few helpful hints on skin care.

This book falls in neither category. Its emphasis is on *skin care: how to keep skin healthy and how to make and keep it attractive.* This book's approach is positive, based on both a medical and industrial background. It expresses my own experience, derived from scientific fact, years of service in the private practice and teaching of dermatology and direct involvement with the research and development of cosmetics and toiletries. A certain amount of bias has been impossible to avoid. Even the telephone directory is weighted in favor of the front end of the alphabet.

Written for men and women of all ages, an occasional section of this book directs information to a specific age group or sex. For example, the male reader's attention may be initially attracted to the section on grooming aids for men. This topic is gaining in popularity, and the products available are rapidly increasing in number. However, achieving healthier, younger-looking skin and learning to complement it with cosmetics requires the fundamental knowledge you will acquire from the many chapters of universal interest.

I hope my opinions are attractive enough for you to want to adapt them to your personal needs. You may find it disturbing, and you may also find it refreshing, to replace your familiar notions and habits with something new and different. If your personal physician's recommendations and mine differ here and there do not fret. This is not at all unusual. There is an old expression: "When two physicians get together, you are sure to get three opinions." If that third opinion is your own, once the physicians have explained themselves, all well and good. For, after all, a lively dialogue is precisely what a useful book is all about.

Many friends, colleagues, and associates proffered aid and encouragement in the preparation of this manuscript. For this I am grateful. The burden of assembling technical details was considerably lightened by the helpful contributions of Mrs. Lillian Dunn Alper (nail care), Lou Burris (hair coloring), Harry Cuttler (fragrance), Mel Kamen (soap), Stan Lawrence (make-up), Dr. D. L. Opdyke (pharmacology), and William Perlberg (shampoo).

EARLE W. BRAUER, M.D.

Bluff Point
Westport, Conn.
November 15, 1968

CONTENTS

YOUR SKIN AND HAIR

INTRODUCTION: I
THE CHARACTERISTICS OF THE SKIN

The color, texture, aging characteristics and many other aspects of skin, hair and nails are inherited from our forebears. When nature has been unkind we can compensate with proper skin care.

Enter a room, a bus, or an elevator, greet a friend or glance at a total stranger. Such simple and basic events are repeated dozens of times every day. Yet during these often fleeting encounters a whole range of impressions is registered on centers of perception—yours and other people's. Somewhere between the speed of light and the blink of an eye, physical appearance, facial expression and various associated colors impress themselves on the consciousness. Sound (such as speech and laughter) and odor join a moment later. But an instant impression of some kind—good, bad, flattering, startling, disappointing or sympathetic—is created by everyone upon everyone.

Although we tend to consider first impressions important, happily our evaluations of people frequently do change as we get to know them.

In our fast-moving and competitive society,

it is not enough merely to present a bland picture of personal tidiness. It is imperative that personal appearance be as attractive as possible. The clothing you wear, the colors you select, your posture and your speech, all are important to your overall appearance; but basic to these factors is the canvas on which you must create your personal portrait, day after day, year after year, for the rest of your life. That canvas is your skin.

Beauty and attractiveness are not the same thing. A beautiful woman or a handsome man can betray nature's attributes by slovenly dress, manner, or make-up. Haven't you often thought of someone: "She could be really attractive if she took better care of herself!"

An attractive woman need not meet the standard for classic beauty. Clever adornment can project attractiveness and charm in abundance.

To work to improve your skin you must know and understand it, how to keep it healthy, its normal changes as a result of aging, climate or occupation. You must learn how to capitalize on your best attributes and what you can do to reduce, hide or correct undesirable features. You must know what will improve, enhance and preserve the appearance of your skin.

Your personal canvas is the product of your heredity. It is worth considering how your ancestors have influenced your skin.

In this age of electronic achievement we may marvel at the accomplishments of the computer, yet the nucleus of every cell of your body is itself a microscopic computer. It was programmed at the time the sperm cell fertilized the egg. The chromosomes in the nucleus carry the messages. At fertilization, every physical characteristic of the human being that is about to develop in the womb of the mother is established: sex, skin color and texture, hair distribution, body configuration, and so forth. Future environment will exert major influences, but the effect that such influences will have is determined by physical characteristics the individual has inherited. Where skin, hair, and nails are concerned, we are able to control the interplay between these two crucial factors—environment and heredity.

For example, skin color and thickness are inherited characteristics. The fair, thin-skinned individual does not tolerate sun well. He burns lobster-red and may not tan at all, building up no resistance to further exposure. Repeated exposure to the sun over a period of years irreversibly damages his skin. It seems to age before its time. Skin cancers may develop. In contrast, the individual who has inherited a darker skin tans easily and suffers less skin damage over the years. His chances of developing cancer of the skin are not as great; other aging effects are lessened. With the Negro, this built-in skin protection functions so well that sun-induced skin cancer is very rare.

If the fair-skinned person will learn to avoid unnecessary exposure to the sun, select an indoor type of employment, remember to use sun-protective clothing and sun-screen creams, then his skin will not only age less rapidly, but the danger of skin cancer can be minimized.

Skin oiliness is also an inherited factor. Persons with less active oil glands may be less prone to develop acne, but more likely to suffer irritation from wind, dust, and chemicals. Any general skin care program must be individualized to take into account these variations.

Hair texture, thickness, degree of waviness, as well as color, are all inherited characteristics. The ability of your hair to withstand the repeated influences of simple grooming or the effects of waving, bleaching or coloring depends to a great extent on characteristics you have inherited.

We are a mixture of the traits of past generations. This mixture, which depends on chance as the chromosome messages from both parents are paired and influence each other, makes us different not only from our parents, but also from our brothers and sisters. (The only exception is identical twins.) What was good for mother, grandmother, or sister, therefore, may be absolutely bad for you.

We turn to the physician, particularly the dermatologist (skin specialist), to diagnose and treat the skin when it is unhealthy. Unfortunately, the time of most physicians is limited; their attention is essentially captured by the immediate problems of disease. They give too little time to healthy skin and less for the patient who seeks advice on how to "dress up" the skin to make it more attractive.

Patients searching for such answers are as much in need of professional help as those with an actual skin disease. Many skin disorders are related to emotional tensions created in patients who believe they look old, that their attractiveness is fading.

A woman naturally becomes concerned when she feels her husband's interest in her is waning, and such agitation can cause medical problems, even skin eruptions. The physician who recognizes this can do more for his patient's welfare by advising her to "Color your hair, dress up your face" than by prescribing tranquilizers or other medications.

This is equally true for both sexes. The average male tends cosmetically to play the part of the unconcerned or reluctant sex. This is only a posture he assumes for the benefit of his peers. The male is becoming more conscious of his person. He is becoming more eager to be pleasing and attractive to those about him, particularly as those about him look less their age!

It is a common error to admire someone's complexion or hair and then to hope to duplicate it for yourself by following that individual's personal habits. It is usually a waste of time and effort. An honest appraisal of what you possess by inheritance is the first step in achieving the particular image you wish to create. Practice a sensible skin hygiene program to keep your "inheritance" as healthy as possible. As fashion dictates, utilize the many cosmetic aids that are available to achieve your purpose.

In the chapters that follow you are offered the opportunity to understand your skin, how it is constructed, how it changes with time and environment and, most important of all, how you can influence these factors to your best advantage.

With motivation and proper direction combined with the abundance of remarkable products and devices that are readily available, satisfying skin care for health, fine grooming, and attractiveness will be easy and exciting to accomplish.

II THE STRUCTURE OF THE SKIN AND HOW IT WORKS

The skin is composed of layers, glands, nerves, and blood vessels. The hair and nails are special variants of the skin itself. Knowledge of these structures and how they work provides the logic to skin care.

A vital organ of the body is a structure that is necessary to sustain life. The heart, brain, and liver are such structures. The skin is also a vital organ. Deprived of fifty to sixty percent of its outer covering, the human body cannot survive.

The skin is the only vital organ readily visible to the naked eye and conveniently available for care and control. We can observe it, evaluate it, minister to it and reap the satisfaction of watching it flourish. Or, we can neglect it and reap the despair that is sure to follow.

Simply stated, one may consider that the skin consists of two major layers (see SKETCH 2–1): the outer skin, called the *epidermis*, and the true skin, the deeper layer, technically called the *dermis* or *corium*. This deeper layer contains the blood vessels, nerves, and glands. These two layers are firmly connected at a wavy surface. The thickness of these combined layers varies over different parts of the body. Over the palms, soles and back it is thickest; over the face, neck, and particularly the eyes, it is relatively thin.

Look at your own skin surface. Notice the

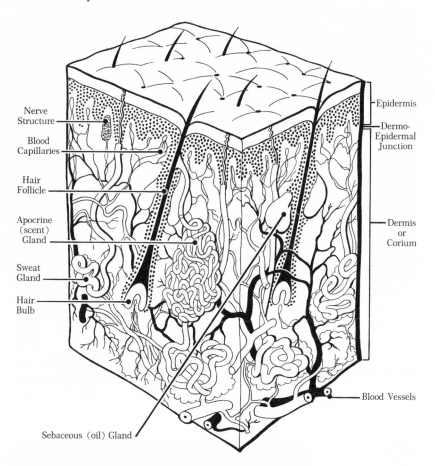

SKETCH 2–1: *A schematic representation of a cube of skin. For simplicity, think of the skin as consisting of two main layers: the epidermis and the dermis. The blood vessels, nerves, glands and hair follicles are all located in the dermis. The wavy dermo-epidermal junction is the boundary between the two main layers of the skin. Note the diamond-shaped markings on the surface and the pore openings for the hair and glands.*

natural markings. These have characteristics for each particular area of the body. Because the hand must undergo many intricate and extreme movements as it opens and closes, its skin is loose and freely moveable. The surface of the thinner skin of the back of the hand exhibits a tiny diamond-shaped pattern with lines over the knuckles. The thick palms reveal crease marks, while the fingertips contain the unique personal "trademark"—the fingerprint. Elsewhere over the body you can see innumerable pinhole depressions commonly called pores which are the openings in the skin surface of sweat and oil glands. From some of these pores you may notice a hair growing. There are crease marks on the face that become accentuated with facial expressions such as smiling, scowling, etc.

All of these surface markings are normal. The degree of prominence may vary among individuals and become more obvious with age. It is this latter association which makes skin markings an undesirable feature. Other things than time may influence these markings and will be discussed more fully elsewhere in this book. It is interesting to note that these markings are less prominent in the obese or chubby individual because thick sheets of fat under the skin tend to fill out the creases. For this reason one will often underestimate the age of an overweight person.

Since the outer skin layer or epidermis is the portion under constant observation and subject to much control, it is necessary that it be discussed in detail. A good understanding of this layer of skin will provide you with the basic principles that enter into the care of your skin.

The outer skin layer, the epidermis, is one of the few unique structures of the body that can and does constantly replace itself. Scratch it, scrape it, peel it off, even cut into it. It heals by replacing itself perfectly, and without a scar, although it may show some temporary color alterations.

Glance at SKETCH 2–2 and focus your attention for a moment at the wavy-lined junction of the two major skin layers. It is at this surface that the epidermis begins. Notice now the first layer of cells. These are the oblong-shaped boxes that are lined up like a string of dominoes. Each has a circular central portion which is the *nucleus* of the cell. Each cell of the body is a living structure in itself. The nucleus is the center of this life—the power structure and command post! Cell division, the ability of the unit to reproduce itself, takes place from the nucleus. Unfortunately, not all cells of the body can reproduce themselves, for example, brain and heart-muscle cells. Once damaged they die and are replaced by scar cells which cannot carry out the particular job that each cell is called upon to do.

The job of the cells of the epidermis is to cover the true skin, the dermis, to protect it (and therefore the body itself) in some very special ways. For example, not only does the epidermis prevent vital body fluids and chemicals from being lost to our environment, but it prevents unwanted and even harmful fluids and chemicals from gaining access to the tissues within. We don't get "water-logged" after soaking in a bath, thanks to the epidermis.

To do this job right the cells of the epidermis must constantly replace themselves. The mother cells of the epidermis are the *basal cells*—the

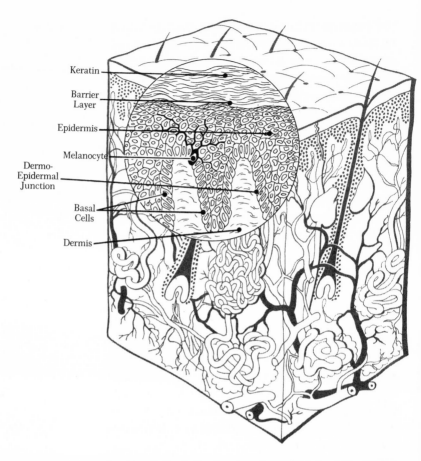

Keratin

Barrier Layer

Epidermis

Melanocyte

Dermo-Epidermal Junction

Basal Cells

Dermis

SKETCH 2–2: *Enlargement of section of upper portion of the cube of skin to reveal cellular structure of epidermis and the dermo-epidermal junction. The basal cells divide and migrate toward the skin surface. During this excursion they become "dry," flat, and stretched out. They pile up in dense layers to form keratin, the normal uppermost surface which is constantly shed. A basal cell requires about 28 days to complete its life span from formation to final shedding.*

The melanocyte looks like a squid. It makes the pigment which is deposited in the basal cells and their neighboring cells.

The barrier layer is not a clearly defined structure. However, it has the important function of regulating the fluids lost from the skin and what can be absorbed through the skin from topical application.

oblong ones at the base (wavy-lined junction) or margin and some of their immediate neighbors. These cells divide to form daughter cells which are gradually pushed or migrate upward toward the surface. Notice that as the cells advance to the surface their shape and size change. They appear thin and flat. As the cells get closer to the surface, it is difficult or no longer possible to visualize individual units. They have become long and compressed. No nucleus is seen; the uppermost surface now appears homogeneous, as represented by the lined portion in the sketch.

This process is actually a gradual aging of the epidermal cells, a drying out, which finally leads to the death of the cells. This firmly packed level, as represented by the lined portion, is called *keratin,* and is gradually shed. It takes approximately two weeks for a cell to be "born" and migrate through the epidermis while undergoing certain chemical alteration to keratin. It requires another two weeks to be shed. Usually this shedding is imperceptible. Although cell division goes on twenty-four hours per day, the greatest activity occurs while you sleep, and probably the greatest amount of shedding, too. Much of the "morning dust" found on your bed clothes is made up of you—shed skin. Cells are also shed under the cast that splints a broken arm or leg, but they have no place to go. They also remain stuck together because of the added moisture under the cast. When the cast is removed, it is often possible to actually see several weeks of shed cells that can be peeled off the skin surface much as the rind can be separated from a tangerine.

The epidermis itself contains no blood vessels or nerves. Its cells receive nourishment via body fluids that pass between the cell boundaries.

There are, however, several very important structures in the epidermis. One is a membrane-like structure, not readily visualized even with a microscope. It is about one-third of the distance down from the skin surface and is called the *barrier layer*. This structure regulates the degree of moisture loss from the skin to our environment. It also bars entry into the skin of many chemical agents that may be applied or rubbed into the skin surface itself. Later on you will learn the great influence this barrier layer has upon the things we apply to the skin surface. You will understand why some preparations work more efficiently than others, depending upon how successful they are in penetrating the barrier layer.

Another important structure of the epidermis is a special cell found occasionally among the basal cells. It is represented in the sketch as the dark cell with the arms projecting out like a squid. Its special function is to manufacture pigment which is then uniquely transferred to the basal cells and their neighbors via its projections and deposited as granules, mostly as a "cap" over the nucleus! It is this pigment which accounts for your skin color. The more pigment deposited, and the more uniformly it is distributed in each cell, the darker your skin color. These pigment-producing cells are called *melanocytes*.

Sunlight stimulates the pigment-producing cells and results in a suntan. This increase in pigmentation acts as a filter to protect the skin against the burning rays of the sun. When your continued exposure to the pigment-stimulating rays of the sun is halted—as with the coming of fall and winter—the excess pigment found in the cells of the epidermis is gradually lost in the natural shedding process previously described. And with it, you lose your summer tan.

Skin pigment can also be influenced by physical or chemical injury, internal disease, medications, pregnancy and aging.

The True Skin: The Dermis

The epidermis rests upon the dermis or true skin. This is a dense layer of tissue which houses the blood vessels, nerve fibers, and special glands which service the skin.

The dermal cells do not renew themselves constantly, as do the epidermal cells. When injured (such as with a deep knife cut), healing takes place by means of replacement with fibrous or scar tissue. This scar tissue has a poor blood and nerve supply and its skin glands may be absent. Consequently, the epidermis which overlies it is not as healthy. It is thin and discolored (usually more pale than the surrounding skin). The larger the injury or the deeper the injury, the more prominent is the scar that will form. If the epidermis alone is damaged or there is only the most shallow involvement of the dermis, then no perceptible scar will result.

The Hair on the Skin

Except for the palms, soles and mucous membranes, hair is normally found over the entire skin surface.

There are basically two types of hair: the readily visible, coarse hairs of the scalp, beard, armpits, genital areas, and, in some people, regions such as the chest and legs; and the soft, thin, short, and almost invisible hairs that are found elsewhere.

The natural hormones of the body exert a

strong influence over hair growth. At puberty the thin and invisible hairs over the bearded areas of men, the armpits, genital areas, etc., are transformed into the darker and coarser variety. The hormones also affect scalp hair and may account for its loss in some individuals.

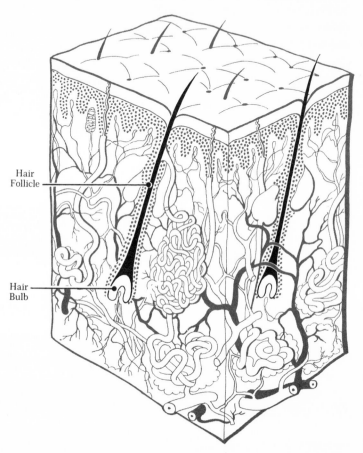

Hair
Follicle

Hair
Bulb

SKETCH 2–3: *Observe that the hair follicle is really an indentation of the epidermis into the dermis. The hair bulb is at the extreme end of the dermo-epidermal projection which has invaded very deeply. The hair bulb cells form hair keratin instead of skin keratin. The hair shaft, as it is formed, pushes upward to the surface and eventually projects from its skin opening.*

The hair grows from a tube of cells that fold down from the epidermis into the dermis (see SKETCH 2–3). This tube of cells makes up the structure known as the *hair follicle*. The cells that line this follicle obviously resemble the cells of the epidermis. They also function by active reproduction in a similar way. The cells that are lower down at the base of the follicle make up the hair bulb or the root of the hair. It is these cells which go through the life cycle very similar to the epidermal cells of the skin. Instead of producing the keratin scale, however, they produce the hair shaft. Chemically speaking, these structures—skin, keratin and hair—are very similar.

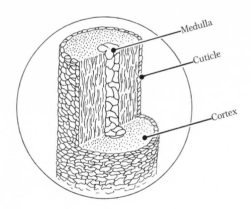

SKETCH 2–4: *A portion of hair filament, greatly enlarged, with a section cut away to reveal the structure of hair keratin. The hair shaft consists of three layers and resembles an insulated wire in its design.*

The cuticle is the hard, glossy, protective outermost layer. If this roofing-tile-like structure is altered, the hair shaft may become fragile when dry; it becomes more porous and will take up larger amounts of water when it is wet.

The cortex contains the pigment granules in its keratin to provide color to the hair. The medulla consists of very special protein substances.

The hair shaft itself (see SKETCH 2–4) is really a filament or wire of firmly packed "dead" cells of unique design. Except at the very base of the hair bulb where active cell growth takes place in association with blood vessels and nerves, the hair shaft is a lifeless structure. A relatively thin but hard outer coating, known as the *cuticle,* acts as a protective sheath about a core within a core, very much resembling an electric wire and its coats of insulation. Once again, pigment-producing cells make and lay down color in the cells that eventually pack together to become the hair filament. Most of the pigment is found in the outer core, the *cortex,* which is just inside the hard outer coating. Variation in normal hair color results from the amount of pigment deposited in the hair shaft and the amount of air which is entrapped between the packed-down cells that make up the hair shaft. In Chapter XI when hair coloring is discussed, these relationships play an important part in the technique of hair-toning and the structural alteration of the hair that is required to produce desired results.

The exact cause for natural curling of the hair shaft is not known. Undoubtedly, it depends on a peculiarity in the architecture of the lower portion of the hair tube or follicle. The cell units are laid down in a slightly off-center manner. This creates a twist or spiral in the hair filament which eventually results in a curl.

Hair does not grow constantly or at a steady rate, but rather in cycles. There is a period of active growth. This is followed by a resting stage. During the resting stage the lower portion of the hair follicle shrivels and the hair shaft it contains falls out. This is the normal shedding process. Following a period of rest, the hair follicle reforms from its shriveled state, enters into an active hair-producing phase, and a new hair shaft develops. These periods of activity, shriveling, rest and renewed activity may each be months to years in duration. Although all the hairs follow this growth pattern, fortunately each hair has its own cycle so that in a healthy state not all the hairs are doing the same thing at the same time.

Particular situations are known that influence hair cycles. For example, in a pregnant woman, fewer hairs than normal are in a resting state (less shedding) and more hairs than normal are in a growing stage. However, shortly after she is delivered of her child the situation reverses itself. More hairs than normal go into a resting stage and increased shedding of hair takes place for several months until her normal cyclical pattern can be re-established. Many women have observed this phenomenon which they falsely attribute to the ether given at childbirth or some equally shocking experience.

It is possible for emotional shock to cause sudden and pronounced hair loss, usually over a small and confined area. The physician calls it *alopecia areata*. It is a coin-shaped area of baldness, usually on the scalp or close to portions of the upper neck, although, occasionally, the bearded portions of the face may be affected. Sometimes more than one area is present and may even appear next to another. This is one of the few types of baldness that is curable because all or most of the hair follicles in a given area are in a temporary resting phase at the same time. It is not difficult for a physician to recognize this situation quickly. While treatment may be given to speed up the return of the growing phase, in most instances, with a little patience, readjustment takes place on its own in several weeks and new hair growth appears (see Chapter XI).

Serious illness, usually associated with high and prolonged fever, some internal medications administered in high dosage, or the accidental ingestion of poisonous substances may also cause a large number of hairs simultaneously to enter a resting phase and be shed. Except in the most unusual circumstances, elimination of the offending mechanism results in prompt return of the hair follicle to a normal growth pattern.

Although it will be discussed in another section of this book, it is probably worth mentioning at this time that various manipulations and procedures applied to the hair associated with grooming, bleaching, toning, etc. may, under certain conditions, cause hair shafts to break. However close to the scalp this may occur, no harm takes place to the hair bulb and no significant influence is exerted on the resting and growing cycle of the hair. Since the average growth rate of the hair is approximately six to nine inches per year, you can readily predict the speed with which broken hairs are replaced. This new hair growth is as healthy as it ever was.

The influence of heredity upon hair growth cannot be minimized. The typical receding hairline and balding crowns of men result from natural and individual hormonal influences upon the hair bulb. More and more hairs enter the resting phase and stay there longer. Eventually the shriveled follicles regenerate only enough to produce a fine, short, and almost invisible colorless hair. Dermatologists call this *male pattern baldness.*

It may take years to cause sufficient hair loss to be obvious. In some persons the progression is noticeable in the late teens or early twenties, at which time it is called premature male pattern baldness. The rate of development is not constant. It is possible for this balding to halt, even remain quite stationary for years before continuing again. The progress, however slow or fast or hesitating, is in one direction only— toward permanent hair loss. Medical science knows no safe and reasonable way to either halt the progress or re-establish hair growth in the non-functioning hair follicles. Methods for improving the condition to achieve significant cosmetic benefit will be discussed in Chapter XI.

The Oil (Sebaceous) Gland

The oil gland, or *sebaceous gland,* is the budlike structure that is connected to the wall of the hair tube (see SKETCH 2–5). It is made up of cells quite similar to the epidermal cells. The appearance of the oil gland is very much like that of a child's balloon. The cells that make up the bulbous part manufacture droplets of oil which are then discharged into the pocket of the gland along with portions of the cells themselves that line the pocket. This is *sebum.* It travels out the neck of the gland into the hair tube opening; from there the sebum finds its way to the skin surface. The oil spreads over the skin surface and coats the hair shafts. While most oil glands tend to use the hair tube as a channel to the skin surface, some oil glands empty directly onto the surface.

The sebaceous glands are in greatest numbers about the face, scalp, upper chest and back. They are found to a much lesser degree over other body surfaces. None are present on the palms and soles.

At the time of puberty, the body's natural hormones begin to function actively. They stimulate the oil glands to a marked degree. This can result in the acne that plagues the teenager.

The oil that is discharged upon the skin and hair acts as a lubricant and also protects the skin from certain environmental factors such

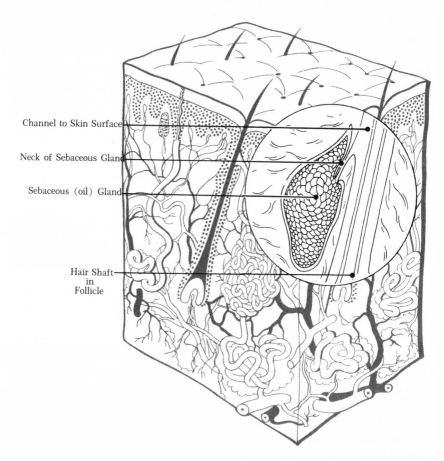

Channel to Skin Surface

Neck of Sebaceous Gland

Sebaceous (oil) Gland

Hair Shaft in Follicle

SKETCH 2–5: *This enlarged sketch shows the sebaceous oil gland which is located close to a hair shaft and actually shares the channel to the skin with it. The oil (sebum) that is made in the gland is discharged through the neck into the common channel and eventually reaches the surface to become deposited on the skin as well as the hair. This mechanism is disturbed in acne.*

as wind, dust, moisture, chemical irritants, and bacteria. It is somewhat of a water-proofing agent, preventing outside forces from entering the skin and important body fluids within from evaporating. The amount of oil deposited on the skin varies with personal characteristics and with climate. Greater oil production takes place in warmer weather.

Surface oil can easily be wiped off and efficiently removed with certain chemicals, particularly soaps and detergents. When the oils are removed faster than they can be replaced; when body moisture is then allowed to evaporate at a greater rate; when outside influences like wind, cold, and dust can gain easy access to the skin surface; then a distinct drying effect occurs and the phenomenon of "chapping" begins.

You will recall in our discussion of the epidermis that the cells migrated to the skin surface, flattened out as they became dry and packed down to form the hard keratin which then, in due time, was shed. If this cell-drying procedure is abnormally speeded up, the corners of the flattened cells tend to lift up from their packed-down position. The edges curl just like a fragment of dry leather. When this occurs the skin is less supple. As you stroke your fingers over the skin surface, it feels rough and spiny because you are encountering the curled edges of the keratin scale. This dry texture is uncomfortable. It tends to itch. A mild inflammation occurs and redness appears. This is chapping. If the process advances, deep splits occur in the skin surface which can be painful, particularly on exposure to the elements or soap and water.

To correct or reverse this abnormal and distressing process, all that is necessary is to permit the deposition of normal skin oils to "catch up"—to overcome the deficit. As the skin ages, the oil glands work less efficiently, consequently, it is easier for this oil deficit to occur; but it is simple to supplement this.

Obviously, the type and manner of skin care will all depend upon age and natural variations, which will be discussed in the chapter on general skin care (Chapter III).

The Sweat Glands

The *sweat gland* (eccrine) resembles a coiled ball of yarn placed deep in the dermis (see SKETCH 2–6). The free end of this ball of yarn, a tube, winds its way upward to the epidermis. From this point to the skin surface (the sweat pore), the tube or *duct* is in a tight, spring-like spiral. The sweat is produced in the deep-coiled portion and is delivered up and outward in a droplet fashion onto the skin surface.

We are born with from two to five million sweat glands which start to function and reach an efficient state of performance before the first year of life. As we grow to adulthood the total surface area of the body increases, but the number of sweat glands does not. Consequently, there are less glands per square inch of skin surface in the adult than in the baby.

Sweat glands are found over the entire body surface except for the lips and isolated areas of the genitals. The palms and soles have the richest supply; the quantity diminishes from head to trunk to extremities, in that order.

Some degree of sweating, although imperceptible to us, takes place constantly. It is one of the important means through which the body regulates its heat. When perspiration evaporates from the skin surface, it takes heat from the body, cools it down so to speak, to the proper temperature. One of the ways the body can lose heat in a hurry is to increase perspiration. If the atmosphere is moist, as on a humid summer

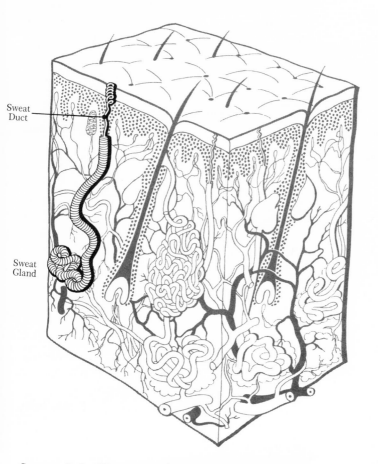

Sweat Duct

Sweat Gland

SKETCH 2–6: *The sweat gland (eccrine) is a balled mass deep in the dermis; its duct transports the perspiration directly to the skin surface through its own pore opening. The terminus of the duct is a peculiar spring-like coil. Blockage of the pore opening may cause "heat rash"; at such times the perspiration cannot be delivered to the skin surface. It breaks through the walls of the duct into the epidermis to cause distressing symptoms.*

day, perspiration evaporates slowly. But step into a breeze, even a warm one, and you immediately feel cooler. This is because the breeze will speed up the evaporation of perspiration which takes heat from the body. This also explains why you feel cool or even chilly immediately after a swim, even on a very hot day. The droplets of water on the skin evaporate like sweat and in doing so take heat out of the body.

The secretion of sweat is promoted by other factors in addition to warmth in the environment, or even body fever. Physical exertion will advance sweating. Pain, fear, anxiety, emotional stress; nausea, vomiting, and endocrine (hormone-producing) gland abnormalities, such as thyroid disease, will all stimulate perspiration. Some medications and foods, particularly alcohol, also induce sweating.

Sweat is clear and watery and contains much salt in addition to a variety of other chemicals in minute amounts. With prolonged periods of marked sweating, as with work or sports in warm weather, a considerable amount of body salt can be lost. Salt is essential for the normal performance of body structures and organs. For this reason it is necessary to add salt to your diet at times of special stress.

Freshly produced sweat has no appreciable odor. It is only when skin bacteria begin to act upon skin surface sweat (or the bacterial decomposition of sweat-impregnated clothing) that a "sweat odor" becomes obvious.

There is another type of sweat gland (*apocrine*), often referred to as the "scent gland," which is more coiled and more complicated than the ordinary sweat gland (see SKETCH 2–7). It is found especially in the armpits, about the genitals, and the nipples. During their production of sweat, these glands also discharge a portion of the cells that make up the gland itself. Consequently, the material deposited on the skin is thick and milky grey in color. Although uncontaminated apocrine sweat is rea-

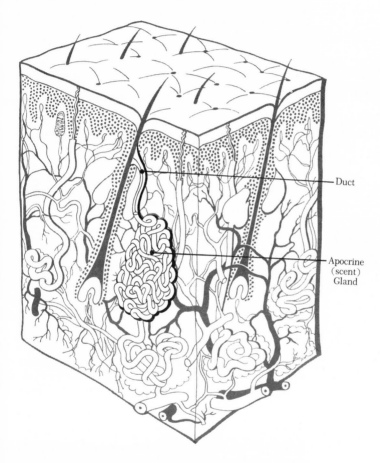

— Duct

— Apocrine (scent) Gland

SKETCH 2–7: *The apocrine (scent) gland is a large densely coiled structure which produces a milky, sweat-like secretion that quickly decomposes on the skin surface to form a characteristic odor. Frequently the apocrine duct joins with a hair follicle to form a common channel to the skin surface. The axillae (armpits) and the skin about the nipples and genitals are rich in apocrine glands.*

sonably odorless, it is quickly and easily acted upon by skin bacteria to produce an individualistic body odor. Some authorities believe that this gland is distantly related to the "scent gland" of animals which attracts the opposite sex. Although the apocrine glands are present at birth, they do not appear to function to any degree until the age of ten. From this time on they become more active and then gradually decline in function after the prime of life.

These glands usually share an opening with a hair follicle in similar fashion to the oil gland. Because of the deep and complicated architecture of this gland, its association with the hair follicle, and its unusual location in areas where skin touches skin, it is subject to infections that may follow minor injury. This simple injury may take place from friction between skin and clothing, or skin and skin. Or it may be the result of a mere pull upon the hair shafts. Careless shaving of the armpits may injure the skin surface. Occasionally an ingrown hair may develop. Such injuries may cause deep and painful inflammation and swelling or abscess of the gland which will require treatment by a physician.

The Nail The nail in many basic ways resembles the hair. The chemical structure of the nail plate is quite similar to the hair shaft. Nail is composed of flattened, dried, packed cells of the epidermis that are generated from the root bed or nail fold that is comparable to the hair follicle. While the hair follicle is a cylindrical tube with the growing portion at the lower end, the nail fold is a flattened channel with one side completely open (see SKETCH 2–8). The growing portion, or root, is also at the lower end and lower sides. The nail plate is firmly attached to its bed. The "moon" represents the newer and thinner nail plate as it has been formed by the nail root. The nail plate is tucked under the skin fold at its base and sides except at the free and most distant edge. The thicker, drier skin that frames the nail plate is known as the cuticle.

It requires about five to seven months' time for a nail plate to completely replace itself, that is, from the time it is formed at the root and gradually pushes itself out beyond the edge of the fingertip where it can be clipped or filed. A toenail grows more slowly. With advancing age the entire process is slowed down.

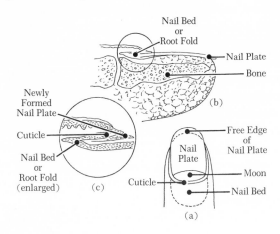

SKETCH 2–8: *Diagrams of the fingertip with emphasis on the nail. In (a) observe that the nail bed beneath the skin extends for a considerable distance beyond the visible nail plate. Figure (b) is an enlarged cross section of the fingertip and it demonstrates how the nail plate grows out from the nail bed. It is similar in design to the hair follicle except that one side (the visible nail plate side) is completely open. Figure (c) is an enlargement of the nail bed to show that it is an extension of the epidermis, just as the hair follicle. Skin keratin, hair keratin and nail keratin are chemically similar, produced by epidermal cells, but possess unique differences for their particular function.*

Like the growing portion of the hair, the nail root is well protected. Injury to the formed plate, as with the hair shaft, will not affect the root or growing portion. Anyone who has ever gotten his finger pinched in a door recalls the sharp pain and hemorrhage beneath the nail plate which caused the blue-black color. With the passage of time, this injured nail plate grew out and was replaced with a normal one.

Injury to the nail root itself need not destroy the nail. It may cause future nails to have a slight vertical ridge, but the nail will continue to grow.

Nail growth can be influenced by local infection or disease processes, by the ingestion of certain medications, and by serious illness and fevers. These disorders temporarily alter the growth pattern to produce horizontal ridging which is more easily felt than seen as the plate grows out.

The nail plate, like the growth circles in the trunk of a tree, can often be very revealing to a skilled observer. For example, if one notices a transverse or horizontal ridge in several nail plates about halfway up the nail, it would be fair to assume the individual suffered an illness or fever about three months previously. It takes about that length of time (three months) for the nail formed during the period of the illness to reach the halfway portion of the nail.

Common nail problems are discussed in a special section on nail care (Chapter XII).

Blood Vessels and Nerves A vast network of large and small blood vessels service the skin to provide the nourishment needed to carry out its many functions and to carry away the waste products that result. The smallest vessels, the *capillaries,* are just wide enough to permit a single blood cell, row on row, to pass through. These capillaries (see SKETCH 2–1, p. 7) reach up to the upper levels of the true skin, the dermis, to the wavy border where the epidermis joins the true skin. Since the epidermis is translucent the network of blood vessels at the dermo-epidermal junction contribute much to skin color. A blush is a sudden widening of the blood capillary tube which allows much blood to enter—and a vivid reddish tint is imparted to the skin. With fright, the reverse happens—the capillaries contract to squeeze out the blood—and a pallor is produced.

There are several kinds of nerve endings in the dermis to signal messages to the brain: touch, temperature and pain. Oddly enough, the common complaint of itching (pruritus to the physician) is poorly understood. There is no special nerve ending to deliver this sensation. It appears that it is carried through the pain mechanism. A lower order or incomplete inflammatory disturbance in the skin, too meager to register as pain, is transmitted through the pain fibers and is recorded in the brain as an itch. The doctor finds it very difficult to treat itch either by ingested or locally applied agents. One of the ways of helping to relieve itch is to overwhelm the skin with another sensation such as cold, heat, or even pain itself. It is often easier to tolerate skin pain than an itch. Many people know they can relieve the discomfort of mosquito bites by pinching the skin or by applying ice or hot water. Extremes of temperature also influence the pain nerve fibers. When the itch becomes pain, it is easier to bear. Many topically applied medications temporarily relieve itch by promoting a cooling or warming sensation on the skin.

It is possible to block all nerve sensations from the skin by the local injection of anaesthetics. These are special nerve-paralyzing drugs that last for many minutes and frequently are used for minor skin surgery.

How the Skin Works

The skin is the first line of defense against our environment. It wards off minor injuries and helps soften blunt ones. By reproducing itself it has a built-in cleansing mechanism. If the skin is stained with some indelible ink or paint which resists all your efforts to wash it off, you know by experience that in a few days it wears off. This is in large measure due to the fact that the stained epidermal cells are shed and replaced by new ones. This self-shedding mechanism also helps us to lose bacteria and other microscopic organisms that normally live on the skin. Such creatures fall into two categories, those capable of producing disease or those that generally do not. Both are present everywhere in our environment and even live upon our skin as well as other portions of the body. Some even contribute to our well-being by preventing the growth of dangerous organisms. Our skin glands help keep the surface of the skin slightly acid to discourage bacterial growth.

Bacteria that merely exist on the skin really need very little encouragement to start to grow and set up an infection. The keratin scale is a good barrier to penetration. Even when it is broken by a scratch or cut, the deeper skin functions quickly to wall off the wound, promote the healing mechanism, and reduce the danger of infection.

The oil gland coats the skin with a thin film which also restricts bacterial growth. In addition, this oil film reduces water loss by evaporation through the skin and offers protection from cold, wind, dust and moisture to maintain skin softness and suppleness.

One of the skin's most interesting functions is its ability to keep the normal body temperature, 98.6°F. regardless of environmental temperature. The brain contains a heat regulatory center that acts as a tiny thermostat. As the environmental temperature goes above normal body temperature, the brain signals the skin capillaries to dilate and become engorged with blood. This makes the skin warmer to permit the loss of heat to the environment by radiation and conduction from its large surface area. At the same time a message is sent to the sweat glands to deliver perspiration to the body surface for evaporation. This also takes heat from the body. If the environmental temperature should keep rising, the above mechanisms are stepped up. As the temperature of the environment diminishes, the system closes down and body heat loss is reduced to a minimum. This is why we are called warm-blooded animals. Fish and reptiles are cold-blooded. They cannot self-maintain their body temperature, but must depend upon the atmospheric temperature for survival.

The nerve endings of the skin act as an early warning system to keep us out of trouble as we approach extremes of temperature or other physical or chemical forces that can lead to body injury.

Constant irritation, such as the friction from

shoes, causes the epidermis to darken in color and to become thick and leathery as a protection from further injury. This is the mechanism that produces corns and calluses. See Chapter XIII.

THE GENERAL CARE OF THE SKIN III

The healthier the skin, the easier it is to make it attractive and beautiful. Its basic care varies with each age group. Soap is a most reliable cleanser. You must learn to select and use it properly. You do outgrow your need for soap. At such times particular cosmetic "treatment" products must be substituted to fulfill your skin's ever-changing requirements.

Caring for your skin involves more than just keeping it clean. You must preserve its good texture and appearance. Caring for your skin means staving off, even avoiding, the drying, thickening, discoloration, warty growths, lines and wrinkles that you have come to associate with growing older. Skin specialists know it is not the mere passage of time that causes all these undesirable alterations in the skin. Rather it is the steady, year in, year out, daily insult of the environment that is to blame. Insult can and should be prevented or certainly reduced. To care for your skin properly, you must have the knowledge and skill to avoid or protect yourself from the everyday hazards that are about you.

If you are past forty-five, man or woman,

take a moment to make the following comparison test. Cut a hole two or three inches square in a five-inch by seven-inch piece of heavy paper or cardboard. Place it over a portion of your skin that is usually covered, such as the abdomen or upper thigh. Make a mental picture of the skin's texture and appearance. Now transfer the cardboard opening to a portion of your freshly cleansed forehead or face. Look at it in a mirror and observe the difference! Both were born at the same time and both have been going around together, but not exactly in the same places. The exposure to the elements helps account for the differences.

The skin is the body's first line of defense, but some areas take more assault than others, and these are the exposed body surfaces such as the face, forehead, ears, neck, upper chest and hands. Wind, dust, grime, grit, sunlight, cold, heat, industrial and household chemicals are only some of the agents which slowly and surely, with persistent exposure, cause alterations in our skin that advance the aging process. Air pollution, with its high sulfur dioxide content, is presently getting much notice for its unhealthy effects upon eyes and lungs. But what about the exposed skin? Sulfur dioxide in the presence of moisture eventually forms sulfuric acid, a compound not known to possess skin-sparing qualities.

It is possible to minimize these atmospheric effects. Diligence and persistence will be rewarded with a more youthful, attractive, and healthy skin.

Cleansing the Skin It is logical to assume that the skin should be kept clean; however, there is no standard method for accomplishing this. Not only does your skin and its requirements change with age, but also with season and occupation. Soap is not the universal skin cleanser. Its improper use on the infant is usually responsible for his summer prickly heat; in the older adult, soap contributes to an annoying winter itch. But for the teenager, particularly with acne, soap may be dubbed the master cleanser.

The action of soap upon the skin is to loosen and remove soil and grime, including body secretions, skin cell debris and bacteria. It is an efficient cleanser that has been known since ancient times. Only fifty to sixty years ago, soap making was a routine household chore. Today, the soap industry practices a most exact science to produce a multitude of products to suit every need and to please the most discriminating tastes.

Soap for bathing and general skin care is readily available in a wide price range from any grocery store, supermarket or pharmacy. These soaps are not all alike. Your selection of the soap that will please you most must depend, as with so many other decisions, upon your basic requirements and how prepared you are to appreciate and pay for certain luxuries.

The important compound known as soap is the result of a chemical reaction between certain fats and strong alkalis such as lye. The curd or flake which results is then treated in a variety of ways to produce a multitude of soap types.

1. MILLED SOAPS.   These are the common soap bars familiar to everyone. The soap flakes are mixed with color, perfume and milled once. The mixture is then compressed and cut into a shape characteristic for the brand, stamped, and packaged. This is a highly automated pro-

cedure which yields millions of cakes of good quality soap.

2. MULTI-MILLED (FRENCH) SOAPS. This is a low-volume process which, in comparison to the milled soap procedure, might be classified as handmade. The initial chemical reaction is carefully monitored to assure the lowest possible alkali residue in the flake. The colors and perfumes are blended with attention to detail; the moisture content is kept very low. Repeated milling of the material takes place before molding into bars. This technic produces a steadfast bar of soap with an extremely fine texture and bouquet that lasts throughout the life of the bar. Quality is built into the bar as in a fine garment. It is understandable that its cost must be greater.

3. WHITE FLOATING SOAP BAR. This soap mixture is prepared with much moisture and no milling is necessary. It is simply molded or extruded into its final form. Since gas is incorporated within it, the bar will float in water. Because of the physical and chemical make-up of such bars, significant soap characteristics are lost rapidly with melting. On storage, the bar tends to lose moisture, change shape, odor, and even discolor.

4. SUPERFATTED SOAPS. These are milled soaps that contain an excess of fatty material. A thin film of oil is deposited on the skin surface to impart a characteristic feel.

5. SYNTHETIC DETERGENT BARS. These are milled cakes containing 100 percent non-soap cleansing chemicals. They possess good foaming qualities and are particularly efficient in hard water areas. Synthetic detergent bars eliminate the bathtub ring. Combination bars are

also made which incorporate true soap in the mixture.

6. TRANSPARENT SOAPS.   These contain 10 percent or more of glycerine and are made from higher and more varied content of vegetable fats. Such mixtures permit better control of the alkaline content and the user is aware of an emollient feel after use. Usually these soaps contain a low level of coloring agents.

7. SPECIAL SOAPS. There are a multitude of soaps and soap substitutes in bar and liquid forms containing medicaments, germicides, abrasive granules, etc. that are available for specific purposes in addition to simple cleansing. Where applicable in the sections to follow, these products will receive particular attention. However, to complete the subject, tincture of green soap is an alcoholic soap solution whose cleansing and antiseptic qualities are of particular value in the care of wounds and other surgical requirements. It is not recommended for general skin care.

In cleansing efficiency all soaps rate very high, regardless of their cost. It probably requires a little more rinsing with water to complete the job when synthetic detergents replace the true soaps in a cleansing bar.

When a rich, full lather is desired, the multimilled (french) soaps are far superior to other types. The synthetic bar is a good second best.

For pleasantness of feel, the sensation that is noted as the moistened bar and/or its lather is applied to the skin, the transparent glycerine soap rates supreme.

If you demand the best possible fragrance performance from your bar of soap, uniformity that is duplicated with each use and will not fade as the cake diminishes in size, then your choice must be a french-milled bar.

There are many features which may dictate your selection: bar size, shape, color, disintegration (melting) speed, type of fragrance, and economy.

If superior mildness is required, I suggest that a soap with a low level of fragrance be selected. It has been my experience that allowing for differences between manufacturers, the transparent glycerine bar, followed by the french-milled and white floating soap, in that order, afford the most desirable mildness benefits.

The Infant   Let's begin with the infant whose keratin layer (outermost skin surface) is thinner than that of the older child. The hairs are finer and almost imperceptible. The oil glands function poorly and the sweat glands are in abundance. (The newborn infant whose umbilical cord area has not completely healed deserves the special attention recommended by the physician in attendance.) Once the cord problem is over, the infant is subject to limited soil to his body. Milk, foods, and saliva contaminate the regions about the mouth, chin and neck; body waste, the diaper area. The ritual twice-a-day baby bath is to be condoned for the psychologic satisfaction derived by mother and child rather than the skin benefit it may provide the baby. It is my firm conviction that tepid water alone, at this early stage of life, makes the best bath. This is so even in warm weather. I do recommend that just a few times a week scant amounts of a mild soap can be used with a minimal of rubbing with the mother's hand, not a washcloth. This is adequate to cleanse the entire skin surface of clothing fragments, dried perspiration and other skin debris to give the child a fresh odor. Between times water alone will satisfactorily accomplish this.

Even the mildest soap, particularly with rubbing, strips the skin of its natural protective oil coating. The alkalinity this produces disturbs the moisture balance of the skin; it also provides a better medium for the growth of undesirable bacteria. It is amazing how well most infants can withstand this unnecessary assault upon their delicate bodies. In the warmer weather, however, they are usually not so lucky. With repeated and frequent exposure to soap baths, a narrowing, even a complete blocking, of the sweat gland openings on the skin may occur. The perspiration that is formed in the gland cannot be delivered to the surface. It breaks through its channel and into the skin to cause an irritation and inflammation known as prickly heat. *The avoidance of unnecessary soap is the best way to prevent this from happening.*

The diaper area requires special and individual attention. Diaper waste is particularly irritating to skin. A cardinal rule is to change soiled diapers frequently to reduce the time that irritating chemicals and bacteria from feces and urine can be in contact with the skin. Feces that adhere to the skin can be easily removed by gentle cleansing with a soft cloth or cotton ball saturated with an oily lotion. Surgical gauze squares are too coarse for this type of cleansing. If the skin is markedly reddened or shows evidence of a rash, soap should be avoided; however, a water rinse is quite desirable. The diaper area should then be gently patted dry and dusted with a baby powder. Such powders are usually manufactured with a fine-textured talc which may be lightly scented. If skin redness is pronounced, a coating of baby lotion may be applied before dusting with the powder. This combination acts to offer a little more protection for the skin against the next soiling. Cornstarch should not be used as a dusting powder. It is a food substance which can actually advance the growth of harmful bacteria and fungi.

There are many excellent baby lotions and powders that are manufactured. These products are compounded with great care and skill to perform efficiently at both room and body temperatures. Many are especially formulated to provide a genuine protective barrier against diaper soil. Silicone additives are particularly efficient and easy to use.

As the child becomes mobile, crawls and toddles, the skin has many opportunities for becoming soiled; consequently, the need for soap will increase. However, if the diaper area is irritated, the bath water itself should be free of soap. This is easily done by washing the several soiled skin areas with soap and rinsing before placing the baby in its bath.

The Older Child   In the pre-teen years the need for soap to maintain cleanliness cannot be overstated. A daily bath becomes a necessity. As the sweat and oil glands function more efficiently, the skin can withstand the undesirable effects of soap. Nails must be cleaned often for they can be sources of contamination.

From puberty to adulthood (thirteen to nineteen) a major revolution takes place in the skin. It is related to the dramatic changes that are simultaneously occurring everywhere in the body. Body hair becomes darker and more coarse; all the skin's components become larger and function at peak capacity. It is the oil (sebaceous) glands that demand the most attention. Oil in great quantities is continuously being made and delivered to the skin surface. This is particularly evident about the face, forehead, scalp and shoulder areas. Within minutes after cleansing the face, fresh oil can frequently be blotted up by a tissue pressed to the sides of the nose, chin, or forehead. Not only does this film produce a rather uncomplimentary shine on the young man or woman, but as will be discussed in the chapter on acne (which will also include special procedures for cleansing away excess oil), the oil may accumulate and plug up the gland openings on the skin surface to form hundreds of blackheads. These are discolored oil plugs, not soil. The oil which stagnates in the skin opening is eventually acted upon by the air; it then changes color from a cream-yellow to a brownish-black.

Frequent and prolonged face washings with warm lather aided by a washcloth or a long bristle brush, such as an old-fashioned shaving brush, are most ideal. To a lesser degree, oil and perspiration are freely produced elsewhere over the body surface, particularly the armpits and groin. Routine bathing or showering, several times weekly, depending upon need and season of the year, should become a habit with the youngster.

Fungous infections, especially of the toe webs (athlete's foot) occur infrequently in a child. However, as puberty and adolescence appear and advance, the body secretions alter to such an extent that they may actually permit fungi to grow and produce skin disease. The toe webs, groin, and similar areas where skin surface rubs against skin surface, are most likely to become involved. The fungus grows best in warm, moist and dark areas. As body secretions collect in skin folds, the surfaces become soft and boggy. Friction then produces erosions or breaks in the skin surfaces; the natural barrier to infection is lost. The fungus is now "home-free" to cause trouble—ringworm, athlete's foot, jock-itch, jungle-rot, etc.

Therefore, these special areas require careful cleansing, followed by scrupulous drying. Application of a dusting powder, by its absorption of excess moisture, will improve local skin hygiene.

The Young Adult and Beyond Usually, at the time of young adulthood (twenty to twenty-five) there has been a significant reduction in the oil activity of the skin. While for many soap may continue to be an ideal cleanser, for others it tends to induce more drying than is necessary or desirable. This is particularly important over exposed body surfaces such as the face and hands and during seasons of the year when outdoor exposure, wind, cold, sun, dust, etc., causes its own drying and irritation. Efficient removal of soil, grime, cosmetics, etc., with maximum skin sparing can be accomplished with cleansing lotions specifically designed for such tasks. These preparations incorporate mild detergents with emollients to separate soil from the skin with as little loss of natural skin components as possible.

As adulthood advances, cleansing lotions should increasingly replace the conventional soap washings, not only to the face and hands, but also to the neck and upper chest. And as one advances into and beyond the forties, the frequency of soap applications to the body itself, particularly the legs and thighs, should also be reduced. This is especially true in the colder months of the year. In this age group the oil and sweat glands of the body are working inefficiently; some not at all. Soap strips the skin of the essential body oil necessary for simple skin protection and suppleness; this produces dry and uncomfortable skin. Winter itch, frequently experienced over limbs and torso upon removing clothing in preparation for retiring, or immediately after bathing, is a common complaint heard in every dermatologist's office.

In most instances, the cause is directly related to dry skin. Although natural for this age group, it has become accentuated by climate, artificially heated homes and offices which cause an abnormally high amount of skin moisture to be lost to dry room air, and the excessive use of soap to tax the poorly functioning skin glands beyond capacity. The result is an overly dry, generally uncomfortable, and itchy skin.

This is less likely to happen in the summertime when hot, humid air allows the skin glands to catch up with the body's needs. However, the dermatologist is seeing more and more individuals who complain of a summer itch. It is related to prolonged exposure to air-conditioned offices and homes. Conditioned air, which is partially dry and kept in motion, promotes the evaporation of skin surface moisture to make the body feel cool. In doing so, older individuals and those with naturally dry skin are experiencing skin discomfort, including an itchy rash. When such individuals wash with soap indiscriminately, they merely aggravate their problem. Soap should be avoided. If water alone is insufficient to remove soil, cleansing lotions should be used. It is an example of narrow thinking and prejudice to consider that such cleansing lotions are for the exclusive use of women. Men suffer much the same physical difficulty and can benefit greatly from modernizing their stilted routines.

The application of night creams upon retiring is merely an extension of the principles expressed above. These products protect the skin from moisture loss due to evaporation and provide oils and water to the skin to keep it supple and smooth.

The cosmetic industry is pioneering in the field of general body hygiene. Products have been introduced for regions other than the face and hands. When large surface areas are being treated, it is more than ever necessary to create formulations that feel and wear properly. For example, a cleansing cream for the face, when applied to the torso, may be annoyingly tacky under clothing. One prestige cosmetic brand has recently introduced a complete line of products for general body hygiene that is tailored to fit the demands of all skin regions. Other brand names are being introduced to specifically attract the man.

You must understand that as you grow older your skin undergoes normal alterations. Its working parts are less efficient. The ability of the skin to adjust to its environment will also suffer. It is illogical to expect that the same regimen for skin care can correctly serve each period of your life equally well. How can you recognize natural change in your skin?

Reading the Oil Gauge of Your Skin It is important for you to make a reliable evaluation of the present status of your own skin if you wish to embark on a sensible and effective program of skin care. I have been distressed by the general confusion, even among knowledgeable people, that exists as soon as an attempt is made to classify an individual's skin as to its oiliness or dryness. It is possible that we dermatologists are responsible for much of this confusion, for in our expertness, we tend to use terms that seem to contradict each other.

To evaluate the oil status of your skin, first consider carefully the answer to the following questions: Did you ever have acne pimples or adolescent pimples in your teens, in your twenties or at a later age? Did you ever have blackheads or pus pimples in your teens or later in life? Do you ever have dandruff? Do you ever have an oily scalp? Have you ever noticed redness, scaling, or itching between your eyebrows, in the creases at the sides of your nose, or over the front of your chest between the breasts?

If your answer to any of these questions is yes, then you basically have an oily type skin.

From sixteen to twenty-five, your skin is as oily as it will ever be. It gradually becomes less oily, depending on inherited traits, occupation, climate, and other exposure factors. Consequently, you may have oily skin at forty-five, but it must be *less* oily than it was at twenty-five. Likewise, at forty-five your skin is *more* oily than it will be when you're fifty-five!

The face is the best gauge for determining the degree of oiliness that presently exists. The central portion of your face is the oiliest part of your body. This is the area between two imaginary parallel lines drawn vertically from about the mid-portion of the eyebrows in both an upward and downward direction (see SKETCH 3–1). The outer portions of your face, the upper back, chest, torso, upper and lower limbs have diminishing degrees of oiliness in that order. Simple observation of your face may reveal the glossy surface of an oily skin. An easy test is to cleanse your face gently and thoroughly with soap and water before retiring. After blotting dry, do not apply anything for this test. Upon arising in the morning, observe your face closely in a mirror under a good light. If you have an oily skin, you'll see the shiny gloss immediately. If the shine is difficult to perceive, then your skin is not oily. To make certain, take a fresh facial tissue and wipe one half of your face only. Now compare the two sides of your face. If you can easily see the difference in the degree of oil gloss between the two sides, then you have an oily skin. If the difference is slight or hardly noticeable, if the tissue itself has little oil on it, then you have an average-type skin. If you can observe no difference on your face or the tissue, it means your skin is "dry."

A combined type of skin—oily in some areas and dry in others—*does not exist*. An oily skin may be relatively less oily outside the central portions of the face; a dry skin may have some

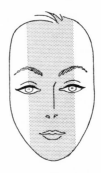

SKETCH 3–1: *The oil gauge of your skin is the central portion (shaded area in sketch) of your face. By observation of this area, as described in the text, you can determine the degree of oiliness of your skin.*

particularly dry areas. But your skin trait is oily or dry, not both on the same face.

An individual with an oily skin may occasionally notice a thin, yellowish scaliness about the nose, mid-chin, between the eyebrows, mid-forehead or even on the cheeks below the cheekbones (the shaded areas of SKETCH 3–1). A slight redness and even a mild itch may be present. This is falsely concluded to be evidence of dry skin.

Quite the opposite, it is evidence of an excessively oily skin. The thin yellowish scaly material is really caked oil and skin debris! It is not dry skin. If proper hygiene for oily skin is followed, this unpleasant problem will vanish. In some few individuals the caking, redness and itch may become very severe and fail to respond to your best efforts. This is called *seborrheic dermatitis*. Your dermatologist can easily and successfully treat it for you.

The Oily Face

The oily face tolerates soap well, and, as will be seen in the special section on care of the adolescent skin, it may be the most ideal cleanser. However, when heavy soil or make-up must be removed, it is very efficiently accomplished with a cleansing lotion. These usually are opaque, often tinted, thick-flowing preparations which contain agents (detergents and emollients) that blend with make-up components to permit their easy and efficient removal. For the oily skin such lotions are heavily endowed with detergents. A soap and water wash may follow; or the application of an astringent lotion, recognized by its alcohol content and usually transparent appearance, may be very worthwhile. This promotes drying and imparts a pleasant sensation by stimulation of the superficial blood vessels and nerves. At your cosmetic counter this product is known by many names, such as toning lotion, freshener, skin conditioner, etc. It will also temporarily shrink down the skin pores.

If you have a very oily face, the type which occasionally shows evidence of caked oil and redness in the central portions (often mistaken for dry skin), the use of an especially strong cleanser and astringent is recommended. These can be recognized as transparent liquids, often colored, which contain much alcohol, in addition to medicaments such as resorcinol to produce the extra drying that is necessary.

The Average Face The average face should be exposed to gentle soap washings only. Therefore, cleansing lotions are recommended as a supplement or actual replacement of soap. This is especially true for the thinner skin about the eyes, ears and neck. The use of an astringent lotion from time to time, particularly before the application of make-up, is most desirable. To assure and maintain good skin surface protection and feel, the additional regular use of a lotion, or cream, known as a moisturizer, which contains an emulsion of easily absorbed oil and water, is important.

The Dry Face Individuals with dry skin should avoid soap. Special cleansing lotions for dry skin have been developed which cause the least insult to the face; however, they remove make-up and soil most efficiently. They incorporate a minimum amount of detergents with a maximum amount of emollients and surface protectants (humectants). Astringents should not be a part of the general routine but their occasional use produces a pleasant stimulating sensation. A moisturizer should be used regularly and often. For dry skin their formulas contain heavier concentrations of oils and humectants.

The categories, oily, average and dry, are the variations of normal skin. You belong to *one* of them. There are no combination types such as oily in one area and dry elsewhere. Your body skin conforms to that of your face.

Age and climatic factors will produce a gradual and progressive drying effect upon your skin. Those who have had the most trouble with an oily skin in earlier years usually have the least difficulty with dry skin in later years. The naturally dry-skinned person is less fortunate with the passage of time.

The important thing to remember is that your skin gradually changes. As it does, you must change the routine for its care. To meet this need, the cosmetic chemist has designed products of many gradations in each type. For the most part, these products are emulsions, combinations of oil and water. The proportions of each will be varied so that the best possible cleanser, moisturizer, night cream, etc. is available to fit your skin.

Oil-in-water emulsions absorb readily into the skin or, if not tissued off, dry easily to yield smooth protective films. Water-in-oil emulsions are basically oily, have little or no tendency to vanish on application and are more suitable for the older or drier skin. You may apply these products directly to your face with your fingers or with a saturated cotton ball. Some may be allowed to dry, others should be cleansed off, even followed by a water rinse. Read and follow the directions that accompany each package.

The facial mask functions as a combination

cleanser and astringent. It is carefully coated on the skin and allowed to dry for many minutes before being peeled off.

Care of the skin is an ever-present daily responsibility. The ritual you establish may, just as with any other routine, become monotonous. You can avoid this by changing to new variations of established products as well as by the occasional use of an elaborate procedure, such as the facial mask. The more diversion you put into your program, the more pleasure and personal satisfaction you will harvest.

The Body Bath

The bath or shower does more than cleanse the skin of the body; it influences mood. It may relax or stimulate. The temperature of the water, its motion on the body, the buoyancy it creates, and the duration of the exposure are important to the effect produced. The claims made for baths at health spas in the treatment of several internal disorders probably result from this feeling of well-being rather than from any inherent quality in the water itself. Some specific skin disorders are indeed benefited by special baths or soaks; however, a discussion of these would be outside the scope of this book.

A warm bath, if time allows, can be a most relaxing experience. However, if the water is hot, it will elevate body temperature. This sets into motion the delicate thermostatic systems of the body. Forced sweating and dilation of blood vessels will occur to throw off heat. The experience, if prolonged for more than a few minutes, can prove physically exhausting. A cold bath can be very stimulating; it can actually reduce body temperature. To conserve heat, the surface blood vessels will contract; this may cause significant strain upon the heart. Consequently, persons with heart disease, the elderly, and the infirm should be cautioned against these extremes of temperature.

Any time-consuming tub-soaking that is desired should be done prior to or completely without the use of soap. Soap in the bath will make the water alkaline. It strips skin of its natural oils in addition to the removal of soil. This stripping will aggravate a dry skin. For strictly skin-cleansing purposes, the shower is more efficient than the bath.

If you insist on bathing or showering daily, it is especially important that you avoid excessive exposure to soap. Refrain from soaping your entire skin surface each time. Confine your soap cleansing to the skin folds, such as armpits, genital areas, and the toes. Clear water elsewhere can provide sufficient cleansing most of the time.

In the colder months, when oil glands work less efficiently, much of the dry skin complaints, particularly itch, can be avoided by the mature person if soap is used sparingly.

In the summertime, when the frequency of bathing and showering increases, excessive exposure to soap can produce heat rash or prickly heat. This is a red, itchy, often bumpy eruption that can be most annoying, regardless of your age. While it may appear anywhere, the neck, chest, upper-inner portions of the arms and regions of the flanks and thighs are common sites. The strict avoidance of soap and the frequent application of a soothing lotion, such as the moisturizer described above in the discussion of the dry face, should produce relief in a few days. Extreme eruptions may require the guidance of your personal physician.

Bath oils deposit a thin layer of oil over the

body surface. In addition to a smooth, rich feeling, this film tends to reduce water evaporation and improve dry skin. These oils also become deposited on the bathtub itself. Consequently, great care should be exercised in getting into and out of such tubs to avoid losing your foothold.

There are many other ways to add to the comfort, enjoyment and relaxation of a bath. The use of "bubble salts," special bath fragrances, and numerous devices such as pillows, table rests, reading stands, etc. need only be mentioned.

In this chapter I have been discussing a group of preparations generally referred to in the cosmetic industry as "treatment products." They are different from the "make-up products" which adorn the skin. These will be discussed in later chapters. As you can see, the treatment products are not offered for the treatment of disease. They are, however, uniquely designed to perform skin hygienic procedures—cleansing, protection and preservation—as efficiently and as safely as possible within the normal, ever-changing pattern of your skin.

The scientific accomplishments in chemistry, biology, pharmacology, physiology, etc. which have advanced medicine in the past forty years have also influenced the field of cosmetic science. If you were ill, you would not want to limit the medications your doctor could prescribe to those in use in 1930! Likewise, in caring for your skin today, you do not want products that bear the imprint of knowledge limited to that which is four decades old. The cosmetic chemist uses modern materials in new physico-chemical systems to yield the best possible products. What was good enough for grandmother in her day is not good enough for you now.

Select your cosmetics with the same critical eye you reserve for your costume and its accessories. In addition to quality you seek certain aesthetics—the pleasure, comfort and satisfaction that accompanies use. No one can measure the importance or value that these constituents hold for you. This is your mystique. Let me encourage you to cater to it within your means.

IV THE SPECIAL PROBLEM OF ADOLESCENCE

The teenager is victimized by his own skin. Acne causes torment to his blossoming personality. There is much he can do to help himself. But he must understand the disorder, the means for its control, and the limitations to the regimen.

The body undergoes a major revolution as it passes from childhood to full maturity. The endocrine system, under the control of the brain's pituitary gland, manufactures and discharges into the bloodstream a mixture of complicated chemicals, called *hormones*. These hormones stimulate body organs and structures to develop and mature during the gradual transformation to adulthood. This chemical mixture which is responsible for all the amazing and desirable changes that take place: beard growth, deep voice, breast development and menstruation stimulate into excessive activity the oil glands of the body which are in great abundance over the face, chest and back. Often crops of distressing blemishes appear: tiny elevations, blackheads, even pus pimples and painful lumps. This is acne. It appears at a most inopportune time.

It is the time when the teenager, boy or girl, is most conscious of and confused by his or her rapidly changing body contours and behavior; there is increased awareness of the opposite sex. This is the age of extreme critical self-appraisal. Anxious to look his best, he may actually be displaying his worst face because of acne. More distressing is the fact that the teenager who is experiencing this outbreak of the skin learns it is unpredictable. There are good days and bad days. He (or she) cannot be at all certain what he will look like next Saturday night. He begins to lose confidence in himself. This can have a serious effect on personality. At such a time in an adolescent's life, a large measure of sound and comforting advice is needed.

Acne and Its Causes

Many factors in combination cause acne. The profuse, irregular, and unbalanced production of hormones stimulates the oil glands to manufacture large quantities of thickened skin oil. The tube-like channel and opening of the oil gland, which is usually shared with a hair shaft (see SKETCHES 2–1 and 2–5), narrows at the skin surface. Oil collects in this apparatus; it becomes thicker and its delivery to the skin surface becomes more sluggish. A plug of hardened oil eventually forms inside the gland opening. The oxygen in the atmosphere gradually discolors the top of this plug to a brownish-black. This is commonly known as a "blackhead." Your physician calls it a comedone. It is not soil. If you have ever squeezed one of them from your skin you are familiar with its waxy consistency and the coiled thread of lighter-colored oily material that is extruded. It has a very characteristic, rather unpleasant odor.

The oil gland, under endocrine stimulation, continues to manufacture oil. It cannot pass the blackhead which acts like a plug in the mouth of a balloon. The oil gland, as it fills with oil, continues to expand. It may be felt and even seen as a bump in the skin. Since many types of bacteria are always present on the skin surface, the stagnant oil in the gland is a fertile place for them to grow. An infection or pus-pocket forms. Your physician refers to this as a *pustule*. The infection may invade deeply into the gland itself, resulting in a large, tender, disfiguring red bump—an infected cyst. Frequently, this inflamed cyst will break open by itself to discharge pus mixed with blood and blood components. Because such infections occur deep in the skin, damage may be caused to the true skin (corium) and healing will then result in a depressed pock-like scar.

This entire process may appear in various stages of development over the face, neck and shoulders. The extent of involvement and its severity is an individual characteristic—the result of inherited traits plus the effects of, or a lack of, personal care and hygiene. It is the rare adolescent indeed who passes through the teens without some evidence of acne.

In the vast majority, acne begins at about thirteen and, as the body approaches full maturity, disappears spontaneously by the late teens or early twenties. Some youngsters show evidence of acne earlier than the average; others may continue to be troubled with it even beyond the late twenties. There need be no relationship between the age of onset and the age of disappearance of the acne. Getting acne early does not mean you will get rid of it early or vice versa. No one, no physician, no matter how expert, can predict at what age any one person will stop having acne.

However, it is certainly true that you will eventually outgrow acne. This is small comfort to you and every young and impatient sufferer who wants and is entitled to help and benefit now.

Most young people have reasonably mild acne which can be controlled by simple self-help measures. For the more extensive and severe degrees of involvement, you should seek the special care that an interested physician can provide.

If you are a teenager, you must realize that acne is a normal phenomenon of maturity that is common to your age group. In this sense, it is not a disease or illness which reflects that there is something particularly wrong with you. Many of your friends have the same problem. Acne blemishes do not suddenly appear any more than a flower suddenly appears—even though it may seem so. It takes days of growth within the oil gland to produce the blackhead, and longer yet for the tender red pimple or cyst.

Consequently, there can be no simple, quick method to cure acne in a few days any more than one can grow a tulip in a few days. In fact there is *no cure* for acne at all, other than growing older. But there are many, many things that can be done to successfully *control* acne—subdue it; keep it of such small dimension that you are little concerned by its presence and are content or patient to wait through the years when your acne will disappear by itself.

The Control of Acne

All too frequently, brides, grooms, or their attendants with severe acne have consulted me for some magic remedy to clear their faces for the wedding scheduled for the following Sunday! It cannot be done. It takes a physician, and a cooperative patient, many weeks to improve acne. And, once cleared, the treatment program must be continued if improvement is to be maintained.

The care of acne-prone skin is not a sometime thing. The quicker you accept this, the easier it will be to begin and maintain a logical skin care program that will yield satisfactory results.

Here is a three-point regimen for you to follow.

Diet It has been my experience that it is absolutely essential for success to prescribe a fat-poor diet and exclude certain foods and medicines that contain chemical compounds suspected of stimulating oil gland activity.

Some foods which should be

Eliminate completely all of the following foods:

> Cola beverages
> Crullers, doughnuts
> French-fried potatoes
> Iodized salt
> Nuts, peanuts, peanut butter
> Olives
> Potato chips
> Chocolate in any form, including chocolate flavoring
> Canned fish (salmon, tuna, sardines) packed in oil

Reduce intake of all of the following as much as possible:

Fried foods

Fatty foods (pork, pork-products, etc.)

Processed meats (frankfurters, bolognas, salamis, meat loaves, sausages, etc.)

Rich and fattening foods (gravies, sauces, salad dressing, icing, whipped cream, ice cream, etc.)

Shell fish (shrimp, lobster, crab, oysters, clams, scallops)

Eat no more than one average pat of butter (¼ inch thick) per day.

Drink no more than one pint (two glasses) of whole milk per day. If you feel the need for more milk, drink skimmed milk or reconstituted powdered milk as desired.

Broiled, boiled or baked foods are good substitutes for fried foods.

All fruits and fruit juices may be eaten.

Avoid medicine containing iodides and bromides such as found in some headache remedies, certain cough medicines, "cold" tablets, vitamin-mineral combinations and sedatives.

Notice that this diet permits all the lean meat, poultry, potatoes, vegetables, bread, fruit and fruit juices, as well as skimmed milk that is desired. Consequently, there is no reason for you to lose weight on this food schedule unless you fail to substitute permitted foods for those items which are prohibited.

Chocolate in any form is to be avoided, as are also cola beverages. The extract from the cocoa bean and kola nut causes concern, not the sugar. There is no benefit in using sugarless products. You will be pleasantly surprised to learn that most candy and sweets, plain cake and cookies, and soda beverages are not denied to you. In my experience, there are chemical compounds common to salt water fish, shell fish, iodized salt and certain iodine and bromine-containing medications which promote oil gland activity: be forewarned.

Avoiding dairy foods with a high butterfat content such as whole milk, cream, butter and rich cheese is well worth the effort. After a brief trial you will soon enjoy skimmed milk in place of whole milk.

This diet is not difficult to keep; thousands of teenagers have been able to follow it for years with relative ease and satisfaction. A little consultation with the cook of the house as well as the individual charged with doing the marketing will help you over some of the apparent rough spots. For example, pretzels are excellent substitutes for potato chips; leftover chicken, hamburger or pot roast make good sandwiches in place of peanut butter for school lunches; fruit sherbet or ice milk is a far safer selection than a sundae when ordering at the soda shop.

Skin Hygiene

A rigid face-washing ritual must become a daily habit. Since you are experiencing the most oil production of your life, you must increase the number of washings per day and the length of time spent at each session. Any soap will be adequate provided a rich lather is produced and massaged over the face for from two to five minutes. While the fingertips or a washcloth are good, a long, soft-bristled brush (similar to a shaving brush) is superior. The trick is to keep the lather moving for the full washing session before rinsing off. It is the friction of gentle massage that strips the skin of its excess and caked oil and loosens blackheads. Hot water is superior to cold for cleansing purposes; following with a cold water rinse is optional.

No less than two such thorough cleansings should take place daily—preferably on awakening and again before retiring. There are many cleansing products specifically designed for the teenager. Ordinary soaps, special detergent bars, lotions, gels, any of which may contain solvents, tar, salicylic acid, resorcinol, and/or hexachlorophene or similar antiseptic agents are available. Some of these products also contain cereal granules or similar grains to increase scrubbability. All offer something special which may not necessarily match the product's increased cost. There are many medicated, clear, alcoholic-detergent preparations, such as the toning lotions described in Chapter III that may be used successfully. When time or convenience are important, a satisfactory job can be accomplished by cleansing the face with a cotton ball saturated with the lotion. The impregnated cloth cleansing pad is specifically designed for such instances. While all of these possess merit, I am convinced that they should be used in conjunction with a regular soap washing program rather than to replace it. However, let me repeat the most important feature: regardless of the agent used, it is the _regular, routine washing,_ over your entire teenaged oily skin period (years, if necessary) that will bring success.

Skin Drying

The application of a lotion or cream containing one or more medicaments such as sulfur, resorcinol, salicylic acid, etc. will promote drying, if left on the skin for hours at a time. The more frequently and regularly used, the greater will be the drying effects. The face may become

---

slightly red, flaky, chapped—even somewhat tender. Skin that is much involved, with blackheads, tender red pimples, pus pockets, etc. needs the most pronounced drying effect. Round the clock, twenty-four-hour use of a lotion may be necessary. With less involvement, only day or nighttime use may be required. Application to the entire face is best, rather than confining it only to the affected isolated sites.

Girls are encouraged to use non-oily cosmetics to help hide the blemished skin. This will give you much-needed confidence. There are some complete lines of cosmetics formulated with little or no oils that are specifically designed for the teenage girl. Of course, the use of eye makeup or lipstick poses no problem and may be applied as desired.

The overall purpose of the above routine is to produce drying of the young, oily skin. If your face begins to feel taut, slightly chapped, shows evidence of some slight scaling—is even a little tender when the cream or the lotion is applied—then the routine is successful. It is at this point, however, that you may become disturbed by the drying, misinterpret its meaning, become discouraged with the ritual, and dab comforting oils and creams on the face to counteract the drying. Resist this temptation.

Do not be concerned with the drying that is noted. Your skin is not becoming old before its time. If the drying effect is too severe, then the entire routine should be reduced or even discontinued for a few days. Young skin will quickly return to its normal state.

Give the routine at least a two-week trial. Remember that success is achieved by faithful adherence to the entire program. The diet alone, the face washing alone, or the drying cream-lotion alone are not sufficient. It takes all three items as a team to bring satisfaction. Then, as you notice progress, stay with this team to maintain the improvement it has produced. Acne has its ups and downs. Follow through with the treatment team to prolong your good periods and shorten your bad periods.

If you become discouraged, or if your acne is severe, the expert guidance of a physician is required. He can strengthen the basic routine with a wide variety of more powerful medications, some to be taken by mouth. He may add specialized office routines as well to produce the desired results. The extreme and neglected cases are the ones that develop pitted scars. *Much can be done and should be done to benefit your acne.*

I have often been asked by the teenager: "Why is it necessary to make the skin flaky and dry?" Much of the difficulty in acne is a mechanical one. Thick oil stagnates in an abnormally narrowed skin opening; a blackhead forms. By drying and flaking the skin, these narrowed openings are temporarily widened; oil can more freely reach the skin surface. The flaking actually dislodges some small blackheads.

Another question often asked is, "Should I squeeze out blackheads?" This is a procedure best left to the skilled professional. While many small young blackheads are dislodged with the self-help regimen described above, the bigger and older ones require some form of manual removal.

Face-picking by the amateur cannot be recommended. Under a physician's attention, many blackheads can be removed quickly and with little or no discomfort. This procedure does much to improve the appearance of the skin and it causes no damage.

"If I wear my hair in bangs over my forehead, does it cause the skin to break out?" In my opinion, *no!* Hair combed over the forehead or touching the face does not cause acne blemishes to appear. The youngster with oily skin or acne also has an oily scalp and probably dandruff. Regular shampoos are recommended as discussed in the chapter on hair. The skin of the forehead should be treated in the same manner as the face. If bangs are fashionable, they may actually serve a useful purpose. They may hide from view blemishes that appear on the forehead.

THE SPECIAL PROBLEM   V
OF AGING

The skin need not be as old as it appears. Most effects of aging are caused by exposure to our environment rather than by the passing of years. Many of these undesirable effects can be avoided; some can be successfully eradicated.

Maturing is the attainment of knowledge, the development of skills, the cultivation of a storehouse of experience, the acquisition of countless tangibles and intangibles. It is living—and it should be pleasurable.

You can also measure maturing on a clock whose face is marked off to register the passage of time by alteration of attractive physical attributes: the appearance of wrinkle lines, sagging flesh, discolored, uneven, and warty skin; the absence of scalp hair or its change to mousy greyness; the acquisition of coarse, dark, unattractive hair on the face, about the lips, nose and elsewhere; the loss of luster to the eyes; the diminution in the power of sight and hearing. This is aging—and it may not be pleasurable.

As these and many other signs of aging appear, you must cope with and even conquer them because you are going to live longer with them. In 1925 the average American lived to be fifty-nine years of age; at present, he lives to be over seventy.

It is startling, however, to realize that the seventy-year-old of today is actually younger than the fifty-nine-year-old American of 1925. Guaranteed income and medical insurance programs, such as retirement funds and social security benefits, provide a population of financially independent senior citizens with the physical stamina to match their emotional drive to enjoy life. The man or woman retiring at sixty-five today can look forward to thirteen to sixteen years of an extended vacation. If it is true that you are as old as you feel, it must also be true that looking younger makes you feel younger. We humans thrive on social contacts —the pleasure of companionship and the exposure to others. If you look your best, you will more fully enjoy this period of your life. There are many things within easy reach to help you accomplish this.

What causes aging? The precise answer to that question remains elusive. Although scientists are busily engaged in studying this problem, to date they have succeeded in identifying, measuring and tabulating many pertinent, but, for the most part, isolated and disconnected concepts. It remains for future work, probably not too far distant, to connect up these observations, much like the parts of a jigsaw puzzle, at which time a reasonable answer will evolve.

Living tissue, unlike a piece of machinery, has the ability to repair and even replace itself. This ability is influenced by inherited factors, the actual age of the tissue itself, and the extent of wear and tear it receives. All these factors together contribute, for example, to the appearance of your skin. Elsewhere I have discussed how the functioning of the glands of your skin wax and wane with your age. The skin cells themselves, both of the epidermis and the dermis, are also significantly altered by time.

A great promoter of skin enfeeblement is light —particularly sunlight, natural or artificial. It induces irreversible injury to skin cells which resembles the damage caused by aging. Sunlight actually contributes to the undesirable appearance of aged skin.

In aged skin, the overall thickness or plumpness of all its layers is reduced. The underlying fat and muscle become loose and flabbier. The force of gravity draws the tissue into jowls or saggy pockets.

Compare the sketch of aging or senile skin (SKETCH 5–1) with that of young skin (SKETCH 5–2). The epidermis is somewhat thinner; the wavy margin between it and the dermis is flat-

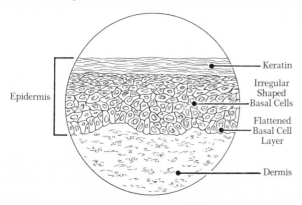

SKETCH 5–1: *Aging or senile skin as seen through a microscope. The epidermal cells are less uniform in shape and size, particularly at the basal cell margin, and haphazardly arranged. Notice particularly how flattened out the border between the epidermis and dermis has become. The tissue of the dermis is also fragmented.*

tened out; the basal cells, which were formerly columnar or cube-like in shape, tend to have a non-uniform shape and arrangement. The cells above them appear piled up in haphazard fashion. The cell contents appear muddy and the cell nuclei shrunken. All this contributes to the dry, slightly scaly, leathery and fine-lined skin seen in aging.

The pigment is less uniformly positioned in the cells to produce the brown, freckle-like areas you may know as "liver spots." In some instances, the normal production and excursion of the epidermal cells from the basal cell layer to the skin surface is so disturbed that actual warty growths develop. Some may eventually result in skin cancer.

In the dermis, the cell fibers and network are also affected. They shrink or become fragmented. You notice it as a loss of flexibility or spring in the skin when it is pressed in; or the sluggish manner in which it rebounds when a fold of skin is held between the thumb and fore-

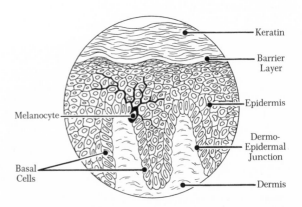

SKETCH 5–2: *Normal non-aging skin as seen through a microscope at same magnification as* SKETCH 5–1 *with which it should be compared. The overall thickness of the epidermis is greater, more uniform in cell content and architecture.*

finger, pulled out a short distance and then suddenly released.

Although these changes are observed anywhere on the skin surface, they are most pronounced, most obvious over exposed areas—face, neck, hands, and arms. There is no doubt that all the features of skin aging are multiplied manyfold by exposure to our environment. The most important single factor in this environment is sunlight. Outdoor workers such as farmers, fishermen, masons, etc. are individuals whose skin represents extreme examples of this exposure.

You can do much to successfully combat the undesirable features of aging skin, particularly the component that results from environmental insult. Begin early in your life, the earlier the better. It is never too late to start, regardless of your age or the present state of your skin.

Basic Care to Spare the Skin

Nutrition

Your diet should contain regular servings of protein from meat or fish and fresh fruits and vegetables in addition to dairy products. Such a simple regimen can easily be maintained, even if you are on a weight reduction program. Fad diets which exclude basic foods should be of short duration only unless supervised by a physician. This is especially important beyond middle age (forty-five to fifty) when the body's ability to digest food becomes less efficient.

Protection from the Elements

Sunlight is an important factor in normal body development. Vitamin D, essential for healthy bone growth in the young, is actually produced by the skin in the presence of sunlight. However, for assurance, particularly in temperate climates, we depend on dietary additives and supplements of vitamin D to fulfill these requirements. When your body has fully matured, the need for direct sunlight is nil.

Prolonged sun exposure, particularly if you have a fair complexion, is to be condemned. The fashion emphasis of a deep suntan is unfortunate. The hazard to your skin from this practice is particularly great. As early in life as possible, establish a practice of sun avoidance: 1) small and gradual doses of sunlight as the summer season begins, 2) constant use of sun-protective creams or lotions to screen out some of the burning rays of the sun, 3) use of clothing, umbrellas, sunshades, etc., especially in unprotected areas during beach and boat activities, 4) reduction or elimination of the practice of prolonged sun-bathing or "frying sessions."

These recommendations are contrary to present custom and practice. They are especially difficult for a young adult to accept. The dividends, however, are well worth the effort. The reduction of sun exposure at any age is worth any effort.

Do not forget about sun exposure in the wintertime, particularly when skiing. The rarified mountain air permits much effective sunlight, albeit for short periods during the days, to get through to the face. Reflection from the snow and ice adds to the hazard. Sun-protective creams and lotions should be used on any exposed skin surfaces.

Excessive exposure of the skin to wind and extremes of temperature, whether warm or cold, should also be avoided. Clothing and the use of skin creams and opaque make-up offers considerable protection.

Routine skin cleansing should be practiced as discussed elsewhere in detail. As natural skin oils are lost with aging, there should be a reduction in the use of soap to minimize skin drying. Body fluids, with few exceptions, are emulsions —water and oils in intimate mixture. The cell components of the epidermis are good examples of this. Cellular shrinkage with age is an oil and water loss. Emollient creams and lotions are emulsions of oil and water. They should be applied regularly to replace fluid loss from the upper layers of the skin as well as to reduce the evaporation of moisture from the skin surface. To a large degree these replacement and protective features account for the pleasant and comfortable feel these preparations impart to the skin.

Night creams for use upon retiring can be formulated to perform particularly well in this manner. They need not contend with the requirements of make-up or clothing and they remain in place for many hours. Their efficiency can be considerably enhanced by the addition, in sufficient concentrations, of female-type hormones, such as estrogens. The key phrase in this statement is "in sufficient concentration."

The amount of hormones necessary in a cream to improve aging skin is of sufficient magnitude also to influence other body tissues and organs such as the uterus and breasts—influences that may be contrary to good health. For this reason the Food and Drug Administration of the United States Department of Health, Education, and Welfare has stringently limited the concentration of such hormones in cosmetic preparations. The permissible limits are so low as to render such products harmless and without value. Any benefits derived from the use of such hormone-cosmetic creams are the result of the cream itself, rather than the hormone contained therein.

The sex hormones are complicated chemical structures that belong to a family of compounds known as "steroids." But not all steroids are hormones. One such steroid, the compound pregnenolone acetate, has no hormonal qualities. It has been reported by some reliable medical authorities to produce desired results on the appearance of the skin. A cosmetic night cream containing this compound *in adequate concentration* has been available for many years.

Special "skin-reviving" qualities have been attributed to some exotic compounds such as mink oil, turtle oil, royal bee jelly, plant extracts, etc. There has been no reliable medical evidence to demonstrate that such substances impart any beneficial effects upon the skin different from the cream itself, devoid of the exotic compound.

Corrective Measures

As the skin ages, its substance, its texture, and its appearance are altered. There is an increase in the number, length, and depth of the fine surface lines. The tissues become loose to form folds and prominent expression lines. Skin color changes and becomes less uniform. The bloom fades.

Removal of Skin Growths

As this occurs, minor birthmarks or moles appear more prominent. They may actually become larger as hormonal balance changes with age, in men or women. Such blemishes detract from your overall appearance. Although you may have considered them quite inconsequential in earlier years, their removal now would produce significant improvement. Perhaps your grandchild has reached out with an inquisitive finger to press one of these fleshy moles on your cheek or chin. Everyone's eye seems to be attracted to them.

The usual method of removal of such growths by a dermatologist is an office procedure; it is simple and quick. A local anaesthetic is injected into the tissues; a sharp instrument is then used to plane down the growth to the level of the surrounding skin surface. In my experience the patient's reaction usually is: "If I had known how simple it all was, I'd have had it done years ago."

Complete healing takes place in ten to fourteen days and the improvement in appearance is most satisfying.

As mentioned previously, aged or senile skin does not work properly. The epidermal cells, in their excursion to the surface, form an incomplete keratin layer. Instead of a smooth skin surface, scaly and warty growths, called *keratoses*, appear. Some are hard and spiny; others soft, crusty, and dark in color. Occasionally, they may fall off spontaneously, or be accidentally rubbed off, only to reform. These unsightly acquisitions to the skin convey an unnecessary impression of age. Some keratoses are more likely to develop into cancerous growths than the surrounding skin. The more fair your skin and the more sun exposure you received in previous years, then the greater the certainty that warty growths will appear on your face, neck, shoulders, arms, and other exposed body surfaces. All of them can easily be removed by a dermatologist as an office procedure.

Following the instillation of a local anaesthetic, a common method of removal is to treat these warty growths with an "electric needle" (a high frequency electric spark), and to scrape (curette) the tissue with a sharp instrument. Due to the simplicity of the procedure, several sites may be treated at a sitting. Healing takes place in ten to fourteen days. Often the scar is imperceptible. The improvement is excellent. As new areas appear, they may be similarly treated to maintain a satisfactory status.

If there are very large skin surface areas affected, such as most of the face, forearms and backs of the hands, more specialized techniques are necessary. Because of the extensive treatment, a short period of hospitalization may be necessary.

One such method is known as chemabrasion. A strong, acid-like chemical is painted on the entire affected surface; this actually destroys a layer of the upper skin. Healthy as well as affected tissue is shed. As the healing process takes places, healthy cells recover rapidly to replace the previous keratoses and skin discolorations. It may take two to three weeks before satisfactory recovery occurs.

Another procedure, known as dermabrasion, actually planes down or abrades the upper layers of the skin by mechanical means. The skin is easily frozen with a refrigerant chemical so that it becomes as rigid as a table top. (Some physicians prefer to instill a local anaesthetic rather than to freeze the tissues.) The surface is then scraped with high-speed rotating wire brushes or burrs to remove the upper layers of skin, normal as well as affected. There is little pain during the treatment; considerable swelling and discomfort may occur in the immediate post-surgical period. Healing takes place in two to three weeks as with the chemical method.

In both procedures described above the resurfaced skin is quite smooth and pink, usually free of discolorations, and much improved over its original state. Of course, neither treatment will prevent the formation of new keratoses. However, by the rapid removal of many dozens of warty growths a healthier and more attractive skin has been achieved in a single treatment. Any isolated keratoses that subsequently appear may be treated individually by simple curettage. Wrinkles, furrows, deep lines and skin bags are not significantly altered by either method.

There has been much recent progress in the discovery and use of special chemical substances that have a particular affinity or selectivity for the warty growths of senile skin. Such chemicals (the most promising is 5-Fluorouracil) upon repeated application, over a period of several weeks, have resulted in remarkable improvement. The keratoses disappear and the skin heals to a smooth and attractive texture. The discomfort and disability which accompanies the use of these drugs appear to be less than that experienced with the usual types of dermabrasion or chemabrasion. In addition, very extensive skin surfaces, forearms, arms, and shoulders which may produce problems for dermabrasion and conventional chemabrasion are easily treated.

Since these new chemicals are particularly attracted by the diseased tissue, the physician can actually see unhealthy areas of skin that were previously too small or too indistinct to be noticed. The application of this medication acts, therefore, as an indicator of future trouble spots. More thorough and effective treatment is therefore possible. It should be emphasized that this method is for the management of the keratoses that accompany aging, sun-damaged skin. It is not a treatment for wrinkles, lines, discolorations or skin sagging.

Yellow-white plaques of varying size may appear about the upper and lower eyelids. These are local deposits of fat particles and known as *xanthelasma*. The tendency to develop such plaques often runs in families and may in some instances be related to the fat particles that circulate in the blood.

Although not necessarily a sign of aging skin, since they may appear in young people, xanthelasma plaques are disfiguring enough to warrant removal.

Such plaques are easily eradicated by either of several procedures: simple surgical excision, destruction by the electric needle, or painting with strong chemicals. Discomfort is minor; the time required for complete healing varies from a few days with surgical removal to about 2½ weeks with chemical treatment. Chemical eradication is a quick office procedure. Although a second or third treatment may be required, no anaesthetic is necessary.

In a later chapter, special (plastic) surgery for the *face lift*—the correction of wrinkles, lines, sags and bags that are the facial hallmarks of aging—will be discussed.

THE SUN— VI
FOR GOOD AND FOR BAD

There is little that is good and much that is bad in modern man's devotion to the sun. The bloom of youth is a constant sacrifice to this relentless god; it pays to do battle with him.

The sun's influence on life is so great that it is easy to understand why primitive man worshipped it as a god. How quickly one's mood improves as the bright light of the sun breaks through an overcast sky! How much stronger the body feels and performs as it is warmed in the comfort of its rays! There could be no staff of life without the sun.

Modern man, through his scientific wisdom, classifies sunlight as a powerful form of natural energy. We all recognize how much our lives depend on it; we all strive to get the most from it. That sunlight injures life is also known, but the medical profession has been slow in translating this into an understandable language for the layman.

A farmer knows, and teaches his son, that too much sunlight even with adequate water can seriously injure the crops. A mother knows and ineffectually teaches her child that a suntan must be acquired slowly if pain and distress are to be avoided. But what this farmer and mother, this son and child, and most of the population don't know, or if they know choose to ignore, is that the same sunlight that is killing the crops is causing skin cancers on the face and hands. The same sunlight that produces the attractive and fashionable nut-brown skin tone, cultivated season after season, will thicken, wrinkle, mottle and age the skin prematurely! Perhaps your reading this chapter will help you get the most that is good and the least that is bad from the sun.

Sunlight is a mixture of several types of radiant energy: visible rays, which account for all the colors of the rainbow and permit us to see and appreciate the world about us; infrared rays that provide the warmth to our environment; and ultraviolet rays which can actually penetrate short distances through the skin to promote chemical and physical effects on living tissue.

There are artificial sources of light which duplicate portions or much of the sun's spectrum. For example: The ordinary household incandescent bulb provides visible light and a small amount of infrared. It gets hot; you can feel the warmth near its surface. The fluorescent light tube is a more efficient visible light source and emits much less heat or infrared rays. Anything hot gives off infrared rays; the heating pad or the hot water bottle are familiar sources of such energy. Heating lamps provide infrared as well as a small amount of visible light. That is why they have a dull red glow.

Artificial sources of ultraviolet rays are generally known as sun lamps. Most small, inexpensive units, oddly enough, provide more visible and infrared rays than ultraviolet! However, there are many efficient sun lamps which can emit light energy that closely duplicates natural sunlight. Some lamps will even reproduce a particular portion or concentration (known as a wave band) of the ultraviolet spectrum for special purposes.

So much of this book deals with visible light—the appreciation of color and form—that no particular mention of it will be made in this chapter.

A measure of warmth, infrared, is essential to life; a little more is necessary for general body comfort. Your body gives off warmth; warmth that gets lost to the environment by direct radiation of your own infrared rays or via the evaporation of perspiration. By managing your environment, such as home heating, use of clothing, etc., you control your body heat loss to provide and maintain comfort.

In exposure to low environmental temperatures for long periods of time, your clothing may fail to protect you from excessive loss of body heat (infrared). The delicate heat-regulating mechanism of your brain will then direct the blood vessels of the skin to narrow down so as to reduce heat loss. Your skin temperature will actually diminish. Its color becomes pale. If the heat loss continues, the brain mechanism demands that your body undergo some physical function to burn food stores to increase heat. The mechanism of shivering is actually a body reflex to accomplish this. If your exposure to low temperatures is maintained, your body will close down blood vessels to portions of your fingers, toes, ears, etc. This can result in frostbite—the actual destruction of tissue due to freezing.

High environmental temperatures cause the opposite effect and blood vessels of your skin widen to carry a greater volume of blood to the skin surface to promote heat loss. Your skin color becomes very red. The ability for warmth, or for infrared rays, to increase the circulation of blood and thereby speed comfort and healing to an area, is readily utilized when a heating pad or hot water bottle is applied to an injured part of the body. A diathermy machine uses radio waves to produce heat in deeper portions of the body for the same purpose.

Effect on Body Tissues Ultraviolet rays, or sunlight (these words will be used interchangeably in this chapter), affect body tissue in several important ways: They actually penetrate into the skin to act upon the chemical systems of living cells. If the exposure is great enough, the substances formed by this chemical reaction cause blood vessels in the dermis to dilate so that the skin becomes reddened. Since large amounts of these substances are formed and stay in the skin for long periods of time (one to two days), the redness persists. Unlike the exposure to simple heat which causes transient redness, this redness does not disappear as you leave the ultraviolet source.

In about four to six hours the dilated blood vessels allow serum (a blood component) to enter the tissues. This causes the dermis to become swollen; pressure and irritation to the nerve endings occur. Like any inflammation, your skin becomes tender to the touch. This is *sunburn*. If the sun exposure has been great enough, the serum poured out by the blood vessels becomes extreme. Blisters will form. It takes several days for your body to heal such damaged tissues.

Meanwhile, the pigment-bearing and -producing cells in the basal layer of the epidermis (see SKETCH 2–2) become stimulated by the chemical reactions initiated by the ultraviolet rays. These cells manufacture, deliver and redistribute pigment to the basal and neighboring cells so that the skin gains a tan color. The epidermis also becomes slightly thicker. All this is nature's reflex for protecting itself, to some degree, from the injury caused by the ultraviolet light. The thicker and more pigmented skin reduces the subsequent ultraviolet light which can penetrate to the dermis to cause the reaction of an acute sunburn. For this reason your skin can better tolerate repeated exposure to sunlight after it has once become tanned. When you are removed from repeated stimulation from an ultraviolet light source, as when summer sun gives way to winter, the cells of all layers of your skin will return to a more normal activity and appearance. In accordance with the usual life cycle of the epidermal cells, the excessively pigmented cells are gradually shed and normal skin tone eventually returns.

Ultraviolet rays are sources of energy of great concern. If the acute sunburn described above covers a large enough body surface, about thirty percent or more, serious illness may occur. This is generally known as sun-poisoning. The chemical reactions caused in the skin can act as body poisons. In large amounts, the body has great difficulty in coping with them—chills, fever, headache, weakness, nausea, shock may occur.

The delicate membranes and tissues of the

eye tolerate ultraviolet rays very poorly; over-exposure results in much discomfort—burning, tearing and sensitivity to ordinary light. Repeated overexposure may actually affect vision.

The fair-skinned individual or the person who does not have the natural capability for producing a skin tan for protection from future ultraviolet exposure runs the greatest risk. He is particularly vulnerable to all the damaging effects of ultraviolet light radiation.

Yet, ultraviolet light can be beneficial. It actually produces vitamin D in the skin which is so essential to proper bone growth in the child. Ultraviolet light is known to improve skin diseases such as acne and psoriasis. Of course, sunlight has always been considered a healer. If you know anyone who suffers from arthritis, you are familiar with his indebtedness to sunlight. In all likelihood the warmth (infrared) and the general feeling of well-being which the presence of sunlight creates is responsible for this reputation.

An isolated instance of acute sunburn is hardly more than an experience in temporary discomfort, minor disability and annoyance at your indiscretion in permitting it to happen at all. However, a measure of irreversible damage to your skin has taken place. Future ultraviolet exposure will produce damage of its own. Damage is added to damage. And the future ultraviolet exposure need not result in evidence of an acute burn. Ultraviolet exposure to your tanned or partly protected skin also causes tissue damage. Although your tanned skin will shield out the redness-producing factor of ultraviolet rays, it will allow through much of the deeply penetrating, damage-producing rays to find their mark.

Although the skin damage produced each time is small, it is damage, added to damage, added to damage year after year after year that produces the major undesirable and unattractive features we usually associate with skin aging.

Medical facts have established that ultraviolet damage advances the aging process of the skin. Reducing ultraviolet exposure will minimize this effect. Suppose one of a pair of identical twins (having medium complexion tone) admired the bronzing effect of a good even suntan; made certain he had one himself each summer; enjoyed being the first in his crowd to have a tan and the last to lose it; lived by the rule—the deeper the tan the better and, therefore, searched out every opportunity for sunbathing. Now suppose the other twin of the pair, living and working in the same city, at the same type job, preferred to avoid unnecessary exposure to the sun; enjoyed outdoor activities in the summer but protected his skin so as to reduce the effects of ultraviolet light; and ended each season very much as he started it, with a normal skin tone.

And now let's suppose that forty-five birthdays have gone by and you meet the twins for the first time. You will observe, with little difficulty, that the skin of the sun worshipper looks older than that of his twin brother. At age fifty this difference will be more obvious; and at fifty-five and sixty it will be startling! Their skin will be anything but identical in areas of greatest sun exposure, such as the face and hands.

The sun disciple's skin is thicker and more leathery; it has more lines. The color is not at all uniform but mottled; it is lighter in some areas and darker in others in a mixed-up crazy-quilt fashion. There are numerous rough spots —warty growths (some of which may eventually become cancerous), particularly over prominent areas such as the forehead, cheeks, nose, and ears. One or two of these rough spots are large enough or dark enough to be seen from a distance. Many tiny veins are also visible on the skin surface. The lips have lost their color and gloss. Their texture is thick and stiff so that cracking is common; they won't stay moist; they have an uneven and warty surface.

This is indeed the appearance of aged skin —much ahead of its time. Side by side, these sixty-year-old twins make a vivid picture. The brother who protected himself from the sun might appear to be sixty years of age to some observers; but by the standards of most, you could easily estimate his age at five or more years less; you might believe him to be but fifty. The sun-worshipping brother, however, will look twenty years older as he stands beside his twin. Off alone, to be kind, you would place him in his seventies; but when he's next to his twin, whose skin has aged normally, *without acceleration from sun damage*, the comparison is too great, and too obvious. As a casual observer they are not twins to you—just a pair of brothers—an older and a younger one!

This accelerated aging phenomenon is taking place—actually encouraged—in millions of Americans, curiously enough in the very society that puts a premium on youthfulness. Although we may choose, in amusing fantasy, to ignore the regular annual appearance of birthdays, we can neither prevent nor delay them. However, we actually can prevent or significantly reduce the skin-aging effects produced by sunlight. Yet, the vast majority of us choose to do nothing about it. What a shocking paradox! But as long as a deep summer suntan is considered attractive and fashionable, and a winter tan is a status symbol, there is little hope in encouraging our population to shun the sun. In all likelihood the very expert—the dermatologist—who is advising you regarding the dangers and future problems you can expect from overexposure to sunlight is himself sporting a deep tan!

Skin Protection

Would you like to begin now to insure your skin from further accelerated aging? Let me describe a convenient, practical and sensible program. Its only objection is that the routine must become a part of your life. You must think about it and practice it, not for a month, a season, or a year, but forever. You must practice it steadily. But it only pays off gradually—inconspicuously at first. The dividends grow better each year as the policy is in force. Like all good insurance programs, the earlier you start, the bigger the dividends. The same problems that exist in "selling" life insurance pertain to this skin-saving plan. Youngsters cannot see the need and do not want it; the older generations understand the need but find it somewhat out of their reach. But whatever your age, whatever the degree of sun damage that presently exists, start now, for everyone can benefit from it.

The more fair your skin, the less its natural tendency to adequately tan on exposure to sunlight, then the greater must be your care and concern in protecting it. The parts of your body that demand the most attention are the hands, forearms, forehead, face, nose, ears, and back of the neck. These sites are exposed to daylight, and therefore some degree of sunlight, every day of your life. Their total lifetime exposure is manyfold greater than those portions of your body selectively uncovered in the summer or for particular activities.

In the summertime, or on winter vacations in the tropics, do not immediately expose your unprotected and tan-free skin to the direct rays of the sun. Sun-tanned skin does have some natural protection but you must acquire it gradually and carefully. The best protection is clothing; it is not always practical. Many sun-protective lotions, creams and gelées (ointment-like) are available at any toiletries counter. Read labels carefully and make your selection with the following considerations in mind: most preparations essentially screen out that portion of the sun's rays that cause the redness. They do permit the skin to tan. Of course, much radiation does reach the skin anyway, but a measure of protection takes place. A very few sun-screening products are more efficient and actually act as a total screen. This means they do not permit the skin to tan at all. Such products are usually opaque in physical appearance—like a very heavy make-up. Since they are available only in a single shade, their use poses problems of cosmetic acceptability. Consequently, they are primarily worn by those individuals under medical supervision for severe sun problems.

Tips on Buying Sun Products   Some sun products, if you will read the labels carefully, make no claim for protecting or shielding the skin from *any* of the sun's rays. They are merely lubricants or moisturizers to help keep skin soft and supple. A popular "sun protective" product of a few seasons ago was just such a preparation. It was used by many in the misguided belief that it promoted a tan and protected the skin. The label, however, made no such claim. The consumer thought it did. Many of my acquaintances read the label for the first time at my urging and were astonished by its wording, or lack of it.

Read the product label carefully and select one that makes actual claims of protection from the effects of sunlight.

With the many types of creams, lotions and gelées available, select one which you personally find most pleasant to use. Products for sun protection must be applied frequently. Read the label directions for use; but remember these are instructions for use under *average conditions.* When circumstances are extreme you must vary your use of the product to suit the occasion. Most products wash off as the skin becomes wet. This is why label directions advise reapplication after swimming. On a very hot, humid day you will perspire freely, even with only modest physical exertion. Perspiration, as it flows down your skin, is also washing off the sun-protective product you recently applied. Toweling off your perspiration from time to time only accelerates and increases your loss of protection.

The sun is stronger at certain hours of each day and on certain days of the year. It is merely common sense that at such times you must be particularly diligent in using the aids you have to protect your skin. You may have purchased a good product, but it can do you no good in the bottle, and very little good unless you consider the many ways you are consciously and unconsciously washing and wiping it off your skin.

Apply the product you select liberally and often to all exposed skin.

Evaluate the sun severity of the day as well as your personal habits. Increase the use of your sun-protective product accordingly, or reduce the extent of your exposure to the sun.

Whether or not you are using a product to promote a suntan, your initial exposure to sunlight should be in cautious and measured amounts. Five sessions of ten minutes each, equally spaced over the course of a ten-hour day are more skin-sparing than one thirty-minute exposure.

Be overcautious. Short, infrequent periods of exposure are safest.

Although the ideal program is one in which your skin does not become tan at all, I am too realistic to expect this restraint from any but the most exceptional individual. There are a few who, for serious medical reasons, must avoid sunlight at all cost. Several uncommon skin diseases and internal diseases appear or become aggravated under sun exposure. In other instances patients may be taking internal medications regularly which render the skin particularly sensitive to sunlight (*photosensitivity*).

Once your usual pale skin tone has changed to a mild tan, you have acquired a small amount of natural protection. It takes very little further exposure to maintain it. The big danger to your skin now is to neglect the need for continued protection. It is a false sense of security, as far as future skin damage is concerned, to believe that because your skin will not redden or blister on further repeated sun exposure, that it is now safe; safe to become as deeply tanned as possible. Sunbathing which produces or maintains *pronounced* tans will just as surely promote all the skin-aging problems you do not want to have in the future.

Maintain your mild tan. Continue to avoid direct and prolonged exposure during the hours of intensive sunlight. Wear the protective cream or lotion of your choice and apply frequently; and as much as possible seek the shade or shelter of canopy, umbrella or brimmed hat. Your dependence upon sun products is especially important at the seashore or on board a boat, for sand and water actually reflect sunlight upward to strike your face.

Don't ever expose yourself unnecessarily to the sun's rays. Clothing gives the best protection; other aids help. Sunbathing sessions are skin-aging sessions.

Probably you have always known all of the above information, including all the rules. But have you been making it a practice to follow these rules? Let me encourage you. Since the real benefits don't appear for years, we all have a tendency to lose interest in a program such as this.

If a deep tan is your passion, it is now possible to have it anytime, at a moment's notice, harmlessly, from a tube. Skin *bronzers* are available. These creams are easily applied, give a natural suntan tone (in either of several shades) and may be washed off without leaving stains or streaks.

Do not confuse these bronzers with the so-called "artificial" suntanning products which enjoyed a short period of popularity some years ago. A few of these, incorporated with a sun-tanning compound, are still available to "speed" the appearance of a tan. They contain dihydroxyacetone, a clear chemical which, when applied to the skin over a period of hours, actually combines with the keratin layer of the skin to impart a yellow-tan color. Unfortunately, this color is rarely normal looking, often appears in streaks, and cannot be washed off. It must wear off with the normal shedding of the upper skin cells over a period of days.

The new skin bronzers impart temporary color only; produce an even, natural-looking tan that lasts several hours and can be easily washed off. This is a good way to sport a tan that has caused no sun damage.

Pigmentation Sun exposure does not always yield an even and cosmetically desirable tan. Occasionally, in fair and red-headed persons, their pigment is not uniformly deposited in the cells of the epidermis. It appears in clusters of cells only so that the effect is one of islands of pigmentation, or freckles. With adequate sun exposure, stimulation of the pigment-producing cells occurs to accentuate the freckling. Actually, the freckling is always present. It is just less noticeable when the contrast between the darker and lighter areas of the skin is slight. As the pigment accumulates following sun exposure, the color contrast increases. It seems as if freckles are forming—when it is just that they are easier to see.

Pigment production can be influenced by hormones. During pregnancy, when hormonal balance undergoes great change, many pigmentary alterations occur in the skin. It tends to darken in particular areas, as the nipples. At such times sun exposure—even winter sunlight—can cause non-uniform pigmentation to exposed skin surfaces, particularly to the cheeks and forehead. This is called *chloasma* or "the mask of pregnancy." After the birth of the child, this discoloration tends to disappear in most women. It may return with each pregnancy.

Birth control pills, to some degree, imitate the hormonal balance that occurs in pregnancy. Some few women who have been taking "the pill" for long periods of time may notice facial pigmentation similar to "the mask of pregnancy."

The use of bleach creams rarely produces satisfying results in diminishing these isolated areas of increased pigmentation. The best bleach creams contain hydroquinone. Daily use for prolonged periods is necessary while simultaneously avoiding the sun. Good results are often lost when exposure to sunlight is resumed. Bleach creams have been reasonably effective in reducing the excessive pigmentation that may follow simple injuries of the skin, such as burns and abrasions.

Dark circles under the eyes are not related to sun exposure. In my experience there appears to be a family tendency to this discoloration; it tends to increase slowly with time. Any puffiness about the lower lids, such as may be caused by fatigue and rubbing the eyes in association with tearing or irritation, accentuates these dark circles because of the manner in which light is reflected. If the puffiness diminishes, the circles will diminish. In many individuals their dark circles remain regardless of the amount of sleep they receive or the care administered to their health. My recommendation to such patients, after reassuring them that the dark circles are of no health consequence, has been to suggest the use of cosmetics to hide them. Bleach creams seem of no value for this problem.

THE SPECIAL PROBLEM VII
OF ALLERGY

The skin can and does develop allergy. Allergic disorders of the skin (contact dermatitis) caused by cosmetics and toiletries are less common than generally believed. Learn how to distinguish products which should be avoided from those that need not be avoided.

It doesn't really matter how you refer to something or by what name or phrase you describe a situation, as long as you are understood by those to whom you are talking. For example, you may call the lovable, curly haired, four-footed pet in your home a poodle. Your family, friends, and neighbors may understand you so that it may never create any difficulty. But if that dog is not a poodle by the standards for the breed, your designation will create a problem for you and for the dog when he is shown to those who really know what a poodle is. In other words, to avoid confusion, we must all talk the same language.

One word that seems to create a lot of confusion is allergy. It means different things to many people. Ordinarily, this would be of small concern. However, in a book of this type, an explanation and understanding of allergic skin mechanisms are most important.

When skin allergy exists, the physician will attempt to identify it for you and help you solve the problem. Many of the dramatic exclamations that I hear of "I am allergic to . . ." are only imagined. They are a self-deduced conclusion based on a series of misconceptions and misinterpretations. Often it is a convenient smokescreen sent up by an individual to provide some temporary or permanent, conscious or subconscious, advantage in a particular situation. For example, your luncheon companion or bridge partner, not to be outdone by the new and very fashionable shade of lipstick you have just shown her, might reply, "I am allergic to that brand!"

I am not at all interested in the game of "one-upmanship." Let us assume your companion really believed what she said. Then it is very possible that she could be unnecessarily denying herself the pleasure of using a particular product or line of cosmetics. In all likelihood she has based her belief on the false interpretation of events in her personal experience. These were matched up with incomplete information from advertisements, product brochures, news items, and/or feature columns; or, perhaps, the experience of others. This chapter is especially directed to you who really want to know what allergy of the skin means and how it affects you.

In an earlier chapter, I mentioned the protective mechanisms of the outer skin surface. Although wonderful in its design and efficiency, this protection has specific limitations. Touch a lighted match or cigarette and you can predict the damage your body surface will experience. The degree of burn, from mild redness to swelling or deep blister formation, will depend upon the temperature of the burning match itself, the pressure with which it strikes your skin surface, and the time the lighted surface is left in contact with your skin. Every person experiencing *adequate* exposure to the lighted match or cigarette will suffer skin damage. No doubt you've played the game of quickly passing your finger through the flame of a candle without sustaining injury. This is because the exposure was not adequate in terms of time. If something had delayed the quick excursion of your finger through the flame, then some degree of burn damage would indeed have taken place.

In very similar fashion, certain chemicals (let's for the moment assume the common agent, turpentine) in suitable concentration, if left in contact with the skin for an adequate period of time, will produce skin damage or irritation in most, if not all, the individuals so exposed. The amount of damage may extend from mild dryness or roughness to itching, redness, swelling, or even blister formation. It will depend upon the concentration of the chemical and the degree of exposure. This explains why turpentine, under specific circumstances, can be safely handled without causing any skin problems.

The Meaning of Allergy

The above illustration describes the simple phenomenon of *primary irritation* which has nothing to do with allergy. In the cosmetic and toiletries industry where skin exposure to its products is great, the use of primary irritants does not exist. Chemicals in this category are carefully and quickly eliminated. However, chemicals capable of primary irritation can be found in common household products: bleaches, cleaning fluids, polishes, solvents, etc. When used with care, as directed, little hazard exists. Of course, there are normal variations in each person's tendency to become irritated from exposure to such products. It is also known that increased frequency of exposure improves the skin's ability to resist irritation—it becomes thicker and more impervious to the chemical.

The skin, on coming in contact with chemical compounds or agents that are not primary irritants, may react in another manner which is quite difficult to understand. It is the mechanism of *allergy*. This interesting medical occurrence will be explained in brief and simplified terms.

Everyone is familiar with the skin eruption that can result from touching some plants. Every geographic area has its particular offenders, such as poison ivy, poison oak, primrose and dozens of others. Since the reaction produced on the skin is via an *allergic mechanism,* it is good for illustrative purposes. Let us consider poison ivy.

You are not born with the ability to develop a skin eruption upon touching poison ivy. You may never, in your entire life, develop such a tendency regardless of how frequently you may be exposed to the plant. You may, however, *acquire* the ability to react to this plant!

Let us assume that on a beautiful warm summer day, a baby of crawling age is taken on a family picnic by his parents to a pleasant shaded knoll. During the course of the afternoon the child (dressed only in a diaper) crawls into the soft green underbrush on several occasions. He is followed, each time, by one or both parents who are barefooted and wearing bathing suits. The following day the mother notices red and itchy areas about her ankles and lower legs. When the eruption becomes more severe on the second day, a physician is consulted. A diagnosis of "plant dermatitis" is made.

Since the only recent exposure to foliage was on the day of the picnic, a cautious visit to the particular knoll establishes the positive identification of the poison ivy plant among the foliage into which the child had crawled, followed by both parents. Although the exposure was the same for each, child and both parents, only the mother developed the skin eruption.

It is necessary now to delve into the past of these three people. The mother, Helen, age twenty-two, was reared in an Eastern suburban area and frequently helped her own parents with gardening chores. When she was about eighteen years old, she recalls having a poison ivy eruption for the first time. Since then (during the past four years) she has had occasional episodes of "poison ivy" following isolated exposures to shrubbery.

The father, Walter, grew up on a farm in New Jersey and never had a poison ivy eruption in his life, although he is certain he's been exposed to the plant many times. He often worked side by side with his brother clearing underbrush. Although his brother frequently developed "poison ivy" and became cautious about working new land, Walter was never troubled by the plant.

The baby has no past. He's several months old and never touched any natural foliage until the picnic episode.

If we were to skin test Helen, Walter, and the baby with the extract from the poison ivy plant, we would discover that Helen's test is positive, while Walter's and the baby's are negative. A positive test means that an allergy is present to the substance tested.

From the preceding story, we may say that Helen is allergic to poison ivy. Her husband and her baby are not! *No one, such as the baby, exposed to poison ivy for the first time is ever allergic to it.* No one, regardless of his age, exposed to any chemical *for the first time* is ever allergic to it.

It is also possible that a person may *never* become allergic to poison ivy, ever in his life, despite repeated and frequent exposures to it. Walter, the father, is just such a person. In like fashion, a person may never become allergic to some chemicals, regardless of repeated and frequent exposure to them.

Some individuals may develop an allergy to poison ivy *after* exposure to it—just as Helen did after her eighteenth birthday. The same could happen with certain chemicals. This allergic tendency may occur weeks, months, or many years after the original exposure. Scientific evidence reveals that it is not possible for an allergic tendency (in this case "poison ivy") to ever take place less than five to seven days after the original exposure.

This means that if Helen and Walter's baby was going to develop an allergic tendency to poison ivy, it would take no less than five to seven days' time from the day of the picnic. This does not mean that the baby would suddenly break out in a poison ivy rash at that time. It means he has now *acquired the allergic tendency.* The baby would then have to be *reexposed* to poison ivy before he would be capable of developing the skin eruption for the first time. From Helen's past history, it took her eighteen years to acquire this allergic tendency!

This variable period of time for acquiring a possible allergic tendency is most confusing to everyone. After twenty-five years of repeated exposure to a particular chemical without any apparent difficulty, a fur-dye worker may experience a skin eruption to the dye for the first time —it has taken him twenty-five years to become allergic to a particular chemical. A young man recently employed at the same task may become allergic to that chemical in a few weeks' time. We know this to be so, but we do not know *why* this is so.

Allergy, then, is an altered or acquired ability of the skin to react to a specific chemical or agent. Not everyone will acquire this altered state. The material or chemical substance which produces this sensitive skin situation is called an *allergen* or a *sensitizer*. These words are used interchangeably.

When allergens cause skin eruptions, they usually produce positive tests when applied (patch test) to the skin of sensitive people. Every preparation, substance, chemical compound, material, whether naturally produced as strawberries, or man-made as plastics, possesses some potential for inducing allergy in some individuals. We can even become allergic to our own body substances.

Allergens are known to have a greater or lesser ability to sensitize skin. This is an important feature because all industries, particularly the cosmetic and toiletry industry, constantly strive to develop and use materials which have the lowest ability to produce a skin sensitivity.

A skin sensitizer or allergen initiates a chemical reaction only when it comes in contact with previously altered (allergic) or sensitized cells.

The biologic reaction which follows is a skin eruption. If the cells of the epidermis (upper layers) are involved, an itchy redness, scaling, bumpiness, or even blister formation may take place. If the deeper layers of the skin are involved, itchy swelling and redness or hives may occur.

Any tissue of the body may be involved in an allergic reaction. However, specific allergens may be capable of affecting or sensitizing only certain tissue. For example, the inhalation of horse dander may cause sneezing or symptoms of asthma in individuals whose mucous membranes of the nose and lungs are allergic to it. The allergic effect may, but need not, even travel through the bloodstream from the lungs to cause the deeper structures of the skin to break out in hives. It would be rare indeed for the horse dander that is deposited only on the skin surface itself (not on the mucous membranes of nose and lungs) to cause an allergic reaction of the asthma type.

The kind of allergic reaction of greatest interest for the purposes of this book is that caused by certain chemicals (allergens) which contact the skin. It is known as an *allergic contact dermatitis* (allergic inflammation of the skin). Through years of experience, the chemicals which possess the tendency to induce allergic skin reactions are well known. All reputable manufacturers whose products frequently come in contact with the skin (such as the clothing and cosmetic industries) scrupulously avoid their use.

The chemical agents which are used in the manufacture of acceptable products possess the lowest ability to induce allergic reactions. Each product is carefully tested in this regard. It is not possible to manufacture anything, or for that matter, grow anything that is completely free of the potential of producing an allergic reaction in some few people in the population.

There is no such thing, therefore, as a completely "non-allergenic" substance; somewhere in the population are a few people with an allergy to that substance. They are but a few out of millions.

The goal of all manufacturers in all industries is to develop products with the least possible tendency of causing allergic reactions in the population. The technical term for this goal is *hypoallergenicity* or *hypo*allergenic products. This word is derived from the Greek prefix "hypo" meaning below or decreased; it does not mean "absence of."

There are some few cosmetic manufacturers who choose to designate their products as "hypoallergenic." I know from my own practice how much confusion this has caused some patients. These are individuals who have suffered from allergic skin reactions caused by products so labelled. With the exception of a few cosmetics which are offered without perfume, these "hypoallergenic" products, with regard to their allergy-producing capability, are *essentially no different from comparable basic cosmetic formulas of other quality manufacturers.*

Allergy to cosmetics is not common. If you suspect that a skin eruption may be related to the use of a particular cosmetic, before indicting it, do the following:

Temporarily discontinue use of the product and allow the skin to recover; this may take several days.

Allergy and Cosmetics

Then return to the use of the product in the manner in which it was intended. If the skin eruption reappears, then your suspicions are well founded and it is best that you avoid that particular product by that particular manufacturer.

However, usually you will find that re-use of the product in question fails to reproduce the eruption. Your suspicions are not justified and you may continue to use it. The original skin difficulty could have been caused by a multitude of casual or specific factors coincidental with, but not caused by, use of the product. It is also possible that after discontinuing the product the original skin eruption persists—which makes it most unlikely that the cosmetic under suspicion is at all responsible. Your problem, then, is not so simple. Skin eruptions may be caused by highly complex mechanisms. Their identification and management require the expert attention of a dermatologist.

A young woman once appeared in my office in great agitation. She had a rather severe eruption about her chin of two days' duration. It was red and bumpy. She immediately volunteered that it was caused by a new make-up product she had bought the previous week.

When I proceeded to question her for specific details, she impatiently replied, "It has to be this new make-up! I'm allergic to it. I felt some 'tingling' near my chin right after I put it on. I only wore it that one time—look at me, my chin. It's getting worse. It even hurts."

This patient did not have an allergy to any cosmetic. What she did have was *herpes simplex* of the chin. It is caused by a virus and is commonly found on or about the lips. You know it as a "cold" or "fever" sore. Sometimes the virus produces its eruption elsewhere than the lips. When it does it may be confusing to the non-dermatologist as well as the patient.

My patient purchased her new glamorous make-up one afternoon for a very important dinner party that evening. Unknown to her, she was also, coincidently, incubating a herpes sore on her chin. The tingling sensation she felt that evening had nothing to do with the make-up. It was caused by the herpes that was developing. The following day the herpes became red and bumpy; it was getting worse. My patient conveniently, but erroneously, matched her skin problem with her new cosmetic.

It takes seven to ten days for such herpes eruptions to heal. I reassured my patient regarding her problem. She was completely won over to my diagnosis when she telephoned me two weeks later. She let me know that her chin was clear and that she was enjoying the use of the very make-up to which she thought she was allergic.

If you have satisfied yourself that a product is at fault, you may find that a similar product in a different line by the same manufacturer or another manufacturer can be used with complete satisfaction. It is a rare individual indeed who cannot be pleased by this procedure.

Some very few individuals have inherited body tissues that are extremely prone to develop allergies. Such people may have asthma-like symptoms or troublesome skin eruptions that begin very early in life. They tend to react badly to many things in their environment—not only inhaled dusts, pollen, etc. but foods and medications taken by mouth, and preparations that come in contact with their skin; their tissues even react to emotional disturbance. This is called *atopy* (meaning "strange disease") by physicians for lack of a better name. When the skin is involved it is called atopic dermatitis. Because such skin reacts almost willy-nilly to so many things, it is very difficult to skin test these patients. Such individuals, obviously, do best with the simplest cosmetics and the most cautious use of soaps and detergents.

Heat, cold and pressure, in rare instances, may affect the skin of sensitive individuals to provoke an allergic reaction of "hive-like" itching on the exposed surface areas.

Sunlight may also produce an allergic response with excessive redness—itching, blisters, etc. This is called *photoallergy*. It occurs on sun-exposed body surfaces. It is caused by chemicals that may be present on your skin or reach the skin from within your body. For example, medications that are ingested may reach the skin and render it particularly sensitive to sunlight. Like most allergies, this can be extremely troublesome. It may take some excellent detective work to uncover the responsible cause.

I am reminded of an attractive young lady who entered my office one day early in February with an oddly shaped, reddish-brown discoloration in the bend of each elbow and on both sides of the neck. It resembled a photoallergic response known as berlock reaction. It is seen, on rare occasions, in the individuals sensitive to an ingredient found in a very few perfumes. Following application of the perfume, the skin site must receive sun exposure—hardly a readily accomplished sequence of events during a New York winter. Careful questioning revealed that it was indeed this young lady's habit to apply a few dabs of perfume to the skin below each ear and in the bend of each elbow; that at Christmas she had received a bottle of an expensive perfume as a gift from a serious suitor, that she had taken the perfume with her on a short winter holiday in Florida from where she had just returned; that she had observed the first signs of the skin discoloration a few days after her arrival in sunny Florida!

In New York the skin discolorations gradually faded and then disappeared completely without trace. To avoid any future difficulty, the young lady switched to another brand of perfume.

In brief summary, it should be repeated that allergies to well-formulated cosmetics and toiletries appear very infrequently in the general population. There is no such thing as a product that is totally free of the possibility of producing allergy in some few people. The avoidance of contact with the offending allergen results in reasonably prompt and complete recovery.

Tracking down the cause of a skin eruption usually requires the attention of an expert physician—a dermatologist. When indicated, he will perform special skin tests—the application to your skin of carefully selected substances and products in suitable amounts and concentration to help in establishing a correct diagnosis. Of the several available skin tests, the patch test is most frequently used. This test tries to duplicate, in minute and controlled fashion, your actual skin contact with substances that may cause allergic reactions under actual conditions of use.

Because hair coloring products may contain dye components to which a small number of users may be allergic, it is necessary that skin patch tests be performed before each use. Such tests are simple to do on yourself; they are easy to read, and an extremely useful guide. The procedure will be described in detail in the chapter on hair.

PRESENTING THE BEST FACE VIII

Make-up for women; grooming aids for men. Emphasis may vary, but the desire to present the best appearance possible is common to both.

The application of make-up is an artistic expression. Each individual creates an illusion upon his personal "canvas." This image is a blend of individual taste and the dictates of fashion. To achieve this effect successfully and efficiently, a variety of materials and products in a broad spectrum of colors is necessary. Your mood and your personality change more rapidly than fashion—often several times a day! The mature executive, male or female, approaches a business conference in a very different mood than that reserved for addressing a golf ball. The young office secretary can hardly be expected to react to the rhythmic noise of her typewriter with the same excitement she will derive from the beat of a dance group. The harassed homemaker's mood and personality is not uniform as she presses on from household chores and taxiing the children, to a theater or a dinner party.

For each mood you select a mode of dress to match. It is equally necessary to match your make-up to mood and dress. Each function of the day demands a particular illusion and effect from you. Excellent and varied products and devices permit you to create the impression you desire in a minimal amount of time and with very little effort. All that is required is a knowledge of the materials that are available and a little skill in their use.

This chapter will provide you with the sequence and the technic for applying basic make-up. It will help you achieve the most natural and attractive effects for both day and evening wear. As you acquire skill and speed in the procedure, you will tailor it to your own taste. You must also be ready to vary the wearing of any make-up as it changes with fashion. When new products are introduced, you will quickly learn where they fit in the make-up regimen and how they may supplement or substitute for others.

Each step in the application of make-up is reasonable; each product in the sequence of events performs an important function. If you have never received competent advice from a make-up expert or a beauty counselor (they occasionally visit department store cosmetic counters), you are possibly very timid in your approach to make-up. To conquer this timidity you must become familiar with the products that are available; you must understand what each is designed to do; and you must acquire the correct material and equipment to do the job properly.

It is as simple as following a recipe to bake a cake. If you don't have all the ingredients called for, or if some of them are not fresh, or if they are folded in in improper sequence, you will not get the cake you anticipated.

Find out what you need in your cosmetic pantry and acquire it. When I say this to some women, their reaction is: "Oh, I have all kinds of bottles at home; I've bought everything and don't know what to do with any of them." I believe these ladies. They are collecting cosmetic bottles just as a boy collects stamps. And some of those half-filled boudoir bottles go back to their high school prom. Too many of the new acquisitions were gifts or the result of purchase by whim rather than logic. No matter how capable or exciting a product may be, it can only perform in concert with others. A good cake is the result of blending matched ingredients that work together. Making up your face requires the same balance.

Making Up

What you must bring to this chapter are: a carefully cleansed skin, the proper equipment and material and an open mind to accept the basic make-up regimen. Leave prejudice and misconceptions behind you.

You must begin with a freshly cleansed face. Follow the cleansing procedure that conforms best to your type of skin as discussed in previous chapters.

Sit comfortably at a well-lighted table which will conveniently accommodate all your make-up material. If possible have two mirrors available. One should be large enough so that you can view your head and shoulders completely from a distance of approximately two feet. This mirror is best mounted to the back of the table or to the wall. The second mirror, for close-up work, can be free standing on the table top, approximately eight inches in diameter, and preferably of the magnifying type.

Very adequate lighting of the room itself, as well as your working or dressing table, is an absolute necessity. Lights may be mounted directly on the frame of the close-up mirror for convenience; however, any good source of direct light may be used. Magnifying make-up mirrors with their own source of direct light are available in a wide variety of shapes, styles and colors. Some even come equipped with hand carrying cases. The two-inch, built-in mirror found in make-up compacts is fine for emergency use and touch-up procedures away from your home. To accomplish an expert-like result, good lighting, good visibility and two free hands are required.

After cleansing your face of soil, you must prepare the skin surface to accept a make-up finish. No painter will apply a finishing coat to raw wood or canvas. He knows that unless he adequately prepares or pretreats the surface (prime coats) with especially prepared material, he will get a poor effect with equally poor wearability. These prime coats act as binding agents for the two dissimilar materials that are brought together in intimate contact for a long-lasting and attractive relationship. In like fashion, your skin, a living and ever-changing surface, must also be made as compatible as possible with the make-up products it will receive. Attention to all these details assures satisfaction in your made-up appearance and provides prolonged wear without "orange" discoloration.

Undermake-up Moisturizer   The first step after cleansing, therefore, is to apply the product known as an *undermake-up moisturizer*. Its purpose is to increase the affinity of your skin surface for make-up, thereby increasing wearability—it produces a film over which the make-up glides smoothly. In addition, it provides a protective layer against the weather. Undermake-up moisturizers are available in several formulations to conform with the degree of dryness or oiliness natural for your skin. As you have learned from previous chapters, your skin status gradually changes with age; consequently, the product that suited you best ten years ago may need revision to meet your present needs. Since the degree of oiliness may also change with seasons of the year (or your menstrual cycle), the undermake-up moisturizer you find most satisfactory in the summer (or certain days of the month) may be too dry for wintertime or daily use. If you know what you want and why you want it, you'll be able to select exactly the product that will give you the best results every day of the year.

Undermake-up moisturizers are also available with color. Like a blending prime coat, this sophisticated refinement achieves a better final coloration. A pink tone will help brighten dark sallow skin; a blue tone should be selected to do this for light sallow skin. If, however, your normal color is florid, with an occasional thread-like prominent blood vessel and you seem to be blushing all the time, then to tone down this coloration, be sure to use a light-green undermake-up moisturizer as a "prime coat." For a natural skin tone, one of the natural shades will produce a uniformly even tone.

Apply the undermake-up moisturizer to your entire face, forehead, and neck—even the ears if they are exposed. Use both hands and blend smoothly, stroking outward from the center of the face. It will dry quickly, imparting a smooth soft feel to your skin.

Foundation   Your face is now ready to receive the major make-up preparation; the one which will create the *basic skin color and texture* you wish to achieve. This product is known as the "base" or "foundation." The color or shade you select must not be markedly different from your normal skin tone; if too light, it will produce a chalky effect; if too dark, it will appear unattractively different. However, previous preparation with a tinted undermake-up moisturizer will permit subtle and effective color-correction of your own skin shade.

The foundation products are available in either liquid or cream form. They are also formulated to impart either a sheen—usually preferred for evening wear—or a matte (unshiny) finish that is more suitable for daytime use.

Apply your foundation with the fingertips. Do not try to do the whole face at one time. Begin with the cheeks, then the nose, chin, ears and neck. Longer strokes are preferred. Carefully blend the sections into each other. Special attention is required at the hairline, around the ears and about the neck. Make-up is most effective when it is not apparent. It must blend with nature to create an illusion of smooth, even, unblemished loveliness. Make-up is least effective when it appears to be competing with nature. All too frequently, a woman detracts from the effect of her make-up because of an obvious sharp line of demarcation between cosmetic and natural skin at the hairline, near the ears or about the neck. If you find this difficult, it probably means you have selected a foundation shade that is too different from your natural skin color; or you may have failed to prepare your skin properly with undermake-up moisturizer to accept the foundation.

The next step is to create the desired surface finish—sheen or matte—and to *set* the foundation for the best wearability with the least need for touch-ups. This can be best accomplished with a translucent powder. You have already applied all the color you need; it is surface finish that you are concerned with now.

Powder Finish

Loose powder is most efficient at this stage. It is available either in frosted texture or the less formal matte finish. Using a puff, the powder is firmly applied to all areas of the face, particularly where the most oil is deposited during the day—such as the nose. Don't rub or stroke the powder puff, as this will cause your make-up to move. Apply it firmly. Loose powder makes the best set. Now blot carefully with facial tissue at the neck and about the chin to avoid rub-off on clothing.

As touch-ups are needed during the course of the day or evening, all you will have to do, in similar fashion, is to apply powder to the areas that require attention. On such occasions, when you are not at home, it is more convenient, cleaner, and far more efficient to use a pressed powder from a compact. Again—be certain to press and not rub to achieve the most effective and long-wearing results.

You are now ready to shape and emphasize your eyebrows with an eyebrow pencil. Notice that your eyebrow is an arched structure that is thicker or broader at its inner portion. It gradually tapers as it extends to the outer side of your face. If you have a uniform oval-shaped face, shape the eyebrow so that the high point

Eyebrows

of its arch is about at the mid-portion of the brow. This will usually correspond to the center of your eye (see SKETCH 8–1a). If you have an obviously narrow forehead which you would like to de-emphasize, begin your brow line lower down, actually closer to the inner corner of your eye; shape the brow so that its high point is over the outer corner of your eye (see SKETCH 8–1b). If, however, you have a wide forehead, the brow line itself should be extended inward; it should begin closer to the nose. The high point of the brow should be located slightly beyond the mid-portion of your eye (see SKETCH 8–1c).

Create a full, natural-looking brow in a shade that most closely matches your hair color. Use short, feathered strokes of the eyebrow pencil

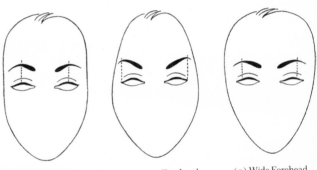

(a) Uniform Oval Face   (b) Narrow Forehead   (c) Wide Forehead

SKETCH 8–1: *The outline of your face will determine the most suitable and flattering shape for you to achieve in fashioning your eyebrows: (a) is the uniform oval outline. The high point of the brows should be at about the mid-portion of your eyes. (b) represents a narrow forehead. The high point of the brows should correspond to the outside of the eyes if you wish to minimize the narrow forehead. (c) represents a wide forehead. The high point of your brows should be located slightly beyond the mid-portion of the eyes to achieve a more uniform appearance of the facial outline. Observe that the length of the brow and its point of origin also varies with each facial contour. See the accompanying text for details.*

to fill in, shape, and color the brow; avoid the harsh artificial appearance of a strong, firm, uniform, pencil line. Be careful not to curve the outermost portion of the brow "down and around" the outside of your eye. This will close in the eye in an unflattering manner.

Eyebrow pencils are available in numerous textures, types and shades to suit individual preference. To achieve an extra-soft natural appearance, eyebrow make-up can be purchased in a cake form for application with a specially shaped brush.

You have now completed the basic steps in the application of make-up. Your face presents a uniform and attractive texture and tone; minor flaws have been minimized or completely hidden. Now you are ready to dress your face in an artistic manner to achieve a particular effect— to match your mood to the day or evening that stretches before you.

Eyeshadow

Begin with the application of eyeshadow. It is here that make-up artistry will afford you the widest latitude for self-expression. Eyeshadows are available in many, many colors; you should acquire a wide selection of shades. Experiment to reflect your personality and to complement your costume. Eyeshadows can be used in stick form for direct application, in creams for use with the fingers, and in cake style for application with a brush. All come in matte or frosted finishes. Here is where you should let yourself go.

Eyeshadow is applied to that portion of skin which you have between the eyebrow and the eyelashes of the upper lid. In imaginary fashion, divide this section of skin into an upper and lower half. Now examine it carefully. If this lower half has a deep, receding crevice as the flexible eyelid curves over the eyeball, then it is best for you to use shadows which are brushed on. The matte finishes will be more satisfactory than the creamy or frosted preparations. With eyes that have this deep crevice, the eyelids fold into deep pleats as the lids open and close. Brush-on shadows are dry; they will adhere smoothly to the skin without caking up in thick strands. If you do not have a deep crevice, then caking up will be no problem. You may use eye-shadow creams or sticks in mattes or frosteds. They will maintain an even surface throughout the period of use.

Shadow should be applied more intensely to the lower half of the eyeshadow area than to the upper half. If you use eyeshadow stick, stroke a band of color directly onto the lid from the inner to the outer corner of the eye; then, with your fingertip, blend the color upward and outward making certain that the deepest color tone is closest to the lashes. The tone is lightest as the eyebrow is neared. To achieve a high-light, an off-white shade can be applied smoothly and in subtle blending fashion just under the eyebrow.

If you prefer a cream shadow, be certain that the skin surface is free of moisture or other make-up. Then press a tiny spot of eyeshadow cream from the tube onto your finger; stroke across the lid from inner to outer portions of the eye, blending and shading off as the brow line and outer portion of the eye area are reached. Remember that the deepest color tone must always be over the area closest to the lashes.

With the cake shadow that is applied with a brush, the same blending application rules should be followed. However, because of the special texture of this preparation, it is imperative that the skin surface be dry and free of any cleanser or other make-up material.

Bright shades will accentuate your eyes to make them appear larger while the muted shades give an illusion of depth to de-emphasize the eye itself. Skillful blending will also help you achieve an effect most flattering for you. If you wish to make your eyes less prominent, then blend color more intensely over a broader area; to make your eyes more prominent, blend for shadow intensity over a narrower area (see SKETCH 8–2).

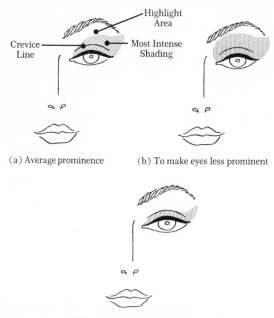

(a) Average prominence   (b) To make eyes less prominent

(c) To make eyes more prominent

SKETCH 8–2: *Eyeshadow shades (color tone) and their blending can help you achieve many flattering effects. For example, a more broad and intense color blend area will make eyes less prominent, as in (b), while shadow intensity over a narrow area will make your eyes more prominent, as in (c). See the text for details.*

There is no limit to the combination of attractive shades you may use in unison to reflect mood or to harmonize with costume. You must only bring to it a measure of freedom for self-expression. The reward is great.

Eyeliner   Eyeliner is usually applied to the upper lid. As with all accent make-up, it experiences many short-lived fads in styles of wear. Its singular purpose is to outline your eyes; to emphasize their shape; and to make them appear larger and fuller. At the same time, eyeliner adds accent to the color of your eyes; it defines your entire costume.

Eyeliner is usually available in three forms:

CAKE: This requires mixing with a little water to achieve proper consistency and depth of color. The liner is then applied with a brush.

LIQUID: Already mixed, this form is also applied with a brush. It produces an intense and more sharply defined line than the cake type. Newer liquids form a clean, long-wearing film that can actually be peeled off the skin at the end of the day.

PENCIL: This is designed for direct application from an easily handled pencil wand; it produces a soft and smooth line. The pencil is the easiest to apply. I recommend it to the beginner, or for those whose hands are less steady.

To simplify the actual application of eyeliner, adjust your free-standing make-up mirror so that you are looking down into it. The mirror should be close to your body; try placing it in your lap. In this position, as you look down into the mirror, your eyelids unfold; more lid area is exposed on which to work. Hold the brush or pencil so that your hand rests on your cheek. Starting from the inside corner of the eye, draw a line across the lid as close to the lashes as possible. As you reach the outer corner, the line should become thinner; extend it a very short distance beyond (less than ¼ inch) the outer corner in a straight or slightly upward direction. If you have pronounced lines or creases at the outer corners of your eyes, draw a shorter line (see SKETCH 8–3).

Use the "flat" of the brush rather than the tip. If you are using the pencil eyeliner, be certain the point is sharpened. A sharpener, manufactured particularly for such pencils, should be kept handy at your dressing table. Moisten the tip of the pencil with a cream or lotion before you use it.

If you are using the cake eyeliner which is mixed with water, it will not line well if there are creamy preparations, such as eyeshadow, over the lid margin. To avoid any such difficulty, powder the lid first.

For daytime use, soft browns are most popular. For evening wear, experiment with black, blue-black, red-black or green-black. If you intend to apply false eyelashes, your eyeliner

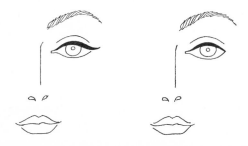

(a) Usual Extension of Eyeliner   (b) Limited Extension of Eyeliner

SKETCH 8–3: *In the average individual, the eyeliner should be extended beyond the outer corner of the eye for a short distance as in (a). Do not extend the eyeliner, as in (b), if you have prominent creases or lines at the outer corners of your eyes.*

should be applied first; after the false lashes have been put in place, touch up the eyeliner.

Eye make-up, particularly the liner, should be removed with care. Water-mixed preparations are easily removed with water; others will respond to a cleansing lotion. There are also available special eye make-up removal pads. Regardless of which you use, be gentle and sparing. The eyelid tissues are thin and delicate. Do not remove and reapply eye make-up repeatedly at one session. If you are experiencing some difficulty with application of the make-up, particularly as a beginner, make do with what you have and try again some hours later. Repeated cleansing over a short period of time, or harsh cleansing, may cause some irritation of the lid surface. I have known women to complain that they are "allergic" to eye make-up when their problem was simply one of irritation from cleansing. They were not allergic at all. As soon as they began to exert care in the cleansing of the eye area, their problem disappeared.

If you wear eyeglasses, they are of little use to you in the application of eyeliner, mascara or false eyelashes; they are actually in the way. If you do not require eyeglasses, but have entered the age bracket of the forties, you are beginning to have difficulty in focusing for close work—especially if one eye has to be closed to receive a false eyelash.

Good light and a magnifying mirror are a great help. Ingeniously designed make-up eyeglasses are now available to further aid you in the ability to visualize the eye that is to be made up. Each lens of these spectacles is of the magnifying type (available in several strengths) and mounted to the eyeglass frame by its own individual hinge (see SKETCH 8–4). This means that if you are working about the right eyelid area, you can free this area for application of make-up by moving the right lens away from the eye. Your left eye has every benefit of its magnifying lens which, in conjunction with the illuminated magnifying mirror, permits you improved vision to perform the delicate tasks about the right eye. When you are ready to work about the left eye, you simply return the right lens to its correct position by closing its hinge; then open the hinge on the left lens to make the left eye area accessible.

Many near-sighted, eyeglass-wearing women and all women over forty who have noticed their vision for close work becoming more difficult, will find this optical system—magnifying mirror and magnifying hinged eyeglass lenses —a tremendous aid. Of course, there are some vision problems that cannot be overcome with this system. However, it may be worthwhile to consult with your eye doctor regarding the feasibility of mounting your own eye correction lenses in the special hinged frames of the make-up glasses.

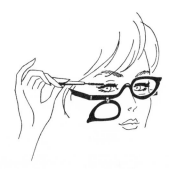

SKETCH 8–4: *Make-up eyeglasses have individually hinged lenses that permit detailed work about the eyes with improved vision.*

Mascara The next step in the sequence of events is the application of mascara to the eyelashes. Mascara colors the lashes uniformly and makes them appear thicker and longer. Even though you intend to apply false eyelashes, an application of mascara at this time will clean off any dust, powder, or eyeshadow material that may be on the lashes.

Mascara is available in all basic shades to match hair color. It is available in special cases equipped with an applicator wand for brushing on or rolling on the mascara in one easy operation, or as a cream. Apply the cream to the tiny brush provided. Then rub the cream into the brush with the end of the mascara tube before stroking the lashes. There are also cake mascaras. These require a little water to mix up to a cream consistency for application with a brush.

Selection of the type of mascara will depend much upon your skill and personal preference. Regardless of the type, however, mascara is applied by brushing the lashes upward and outward. If more color is desired, *let the mascara dry* before applying it again. For greater separation of the lash hairs, make a final brushing with a clean, dry mascara brush. The lower lashes should also receive mascara lightly.

There are mascaras of the case and wand type that contain tiny fibers. With each application of mascara, these become deposited on the lashes to extend their length.

False Eyelashes The most efficient way to achieve the effect of longer and thicker eyelashes is to apply false lashes. They are available in shorter lengths with less density for daytime wear, and in full and extra-full versions for later afternoon and evening wear, depending upon the occasion and the effect you wish to create. Select a shade that matches your own lash color.

Once the false eyelash has been cut and contoured to conform to your upper lid, a surgical-type adhesive, in tiny amounts, is used to make it adhere to the skin surface. Certainly, it requires some patience and skill to master the technique. It is a totally new experience and you are working with only one eye open. But, with the proper light and mirror and with a good-quality false eyelash and adhesive, you will become quite expert after a few practice attempts.

Measure the false lash against your lid margin by holding it with a pair of blunt-tipped tweezers (see SKETCH 8–5). It should be a little narrower than your upper eyelid is wide. If necessary, trim from the outer edge where the lashes are longest. This cut edge must remain the outer side of the false lash so that you will have a permanently designated left and right false lash. Don't mix them up.

To curve or contour the false lash to conform to the natural shape of your eye, hold the false lash at each end of its backing strip, between the thumb and forefinger of each hand; the lash

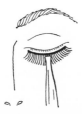

SKETCH 8–5: *Measure the false eyelash against your lid margin; it should be a little narrower than the width of your upper eyelid.*

hairs themselves should point away from you. As you bring the fingers of both hands together, the lash will curve in a horseshoe shape away from your body (see SKETCH 8–6). Now move the edge of the lash in your right hand for a short distance toward your body (the direction of the arrow in the sketch); then move the edge of the lash in the left hand in a similar manner. Alternate and repeat this operation several times. You are actually contouring the lash in a curve that you can match to the natural curve of your eye.

The adhesive you use for affixing the eyelashes to your lid must not be too thin in consistency. It must have good holding power but not dry hard. The attachment of the lash to the skin has to remain flexible for comfort during wear and to permit easy removal. Manufacturers of quality false eyelashes provide good adhesive. If you have any doubt, purchase a

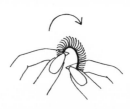

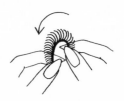

SKETCH 8–6: *To contour the false lash to conform to the natural curve of your eyelid, hold the lash as illustrated above and move your hands back and forth several times before applying the lash adhesive.*

waterproof surgical adhesive which your druggist can recommend.

Dab a tiny bit of adhesive in a thin line along the base of the lash strip. Allow to set for about fifteen to thirty seconds. Press the false lash to the edge of your lid, as you look down into your mirror. This exposes the lid area just as for the application of eyeliner. Never apply the adhesive directly to your lid. If the false lash is not exactly in the right place, use a pair of forceps (blunt-edged tweezers) at one edge of its backing—never by the hairs—to lift and peel it off for reapplication. After a few attempts you will be an expert. The first few times you applied earrings, especially to pierced ears, you thought the procedure impossible, too. But by repeating the effort, you'll quickly acquire the skill and ease that will make the wearing of false eyelashes no more difficult than putting on a piece of jewelry. Wearing the lashes will become second nature; you'll hardly be aware of them.

When the false lashes are in place, reapply mascara to your own lashes to make the two blend together. Then add eyeliner as previously described.

When you wish to remove the false lashes, do it carefully by peeling them off slowly from one edge to the other. Place them to adhere smoothly to the curved surface in their case. This will keep them in the proper shape for future use. At that time the old adhesive is easily removed from the eyelid by peeling it off with a pair of blunt tweezers.

For contouring the planes of the face—to highlight specific areas with a flattering, natural-looking glow, a *blusher,* applied with a soft

Contours and Highlights

brush applicator, is necessary. It can be easily and skillfully applied, even by the most inexperienced or most casual wearer of make-up. Select pink tones for a fair complexion, and peach tones if you have a medium complexion. The deep tones, for those with a darker complexion, provide contouring effects rather than "glowing" effects.

Apply the blusher by brushing from the high point of your cheeks straight out to the ears and into the hairline. This will produce the effect of a natural glow and contour without a line of demarcation. The soft brush permits its feathering directly over your previously applied make-up. Cream blushers that are applied with the fingers are also available but require more skill to achieve professional results.

Lipstick   The mouth is the focal area of facial expression. It continuously projects your mood and personality. Choose your lipsticks with great care for color, creaminess and gloss (light reflectance). You should not want to be known by one lipstick any more than you would want to be known for one dress.

For the most professional results, first use a lipstick brush or a lipliner pencil to outline your lips. This carefully identifies your lips, reduces "bleeding" of color into the tiny crevices about the lips, and improves wearability. Then evenly fill in your lips from either the stick directly or with the flat portion of the brush, using lipstick taken from the stick. DO NOT BLOT! Blotting immediately destroys the attractive texture and gloss. To enhance and preserve this flattering feature, you may, in addition, apply a lip gloss directly over the lipstick.

Remember that the quality cosmetic companies make dozens of shades; most of these shades are available in several categories of creaminess. You should have no difficulty in selecting a lipstick that will feel as good on your lips as it looks.

Lipstick does not change color. If you notice a "bluish-red" color on your lips, it means that it is time to reapply your lipstick.

The color components of lipstick consist of two parts. One, known as the *lake,* provides the shade itself—the color you actually see when you observe the lipstick in its case, or the line it makes as you stroke it on your skin. The other is the *stain*ing component which provides the staying power—that which imparts color to the natural vermilion of your lips. This is the component which does not rub off when you cleanse your lips because it has become an intimate part of your skin surface. (It eventually wears off.) The more stain quality a lipstick has, the better is its wearability between applications.

This second component, the stain, regardless of the shade of lipstick in which it is incorporated, has a bluish tinge. If you observe a change to blue, it means the main color component, the shade which you desire, has rubbed off and only the stain—the bluish portion—remains on your lips. This stain can be pronounced in some few individuals. If it troubles you, there are several things you can do to minimize it:

1. Select a shade of lipstick which has the least staining qualities. The more yellow shades generally have less stain. You can test a lipstick for its stain ability by firmly stroking it on your palm, just below your thumb. Make a line about 1½ inches long. Wait at least five minutes.

Then cleanse the area with a dry facial tissue. If all the color comes off your skin, then the lipstick contains little or no stain.

2. Before applying your lipstick, be certain that the vermilion of your lips (the natural red portion) is free of any dentifrice, cleansing cream, oils, or soap particles. These, being mildly alkaline, may act to intensify any stain capacity of your lipstick. It is best to cleanse your lips with fresh water and wait a few moments for them to dry completely before applying your lipstick.

3. For best appearance, lipstick should be applied frequently during the day. In this way you are showing its true shade, rather than any worn-down color.

The above describes, in some detail, the basic procedure for applying your make-up. It is now your job to vary it to suit your own needs so that it will give you the most enjoyment. Every step need not be followed—but you should know what can be done and what products are available to help you achieve the effects you desire. However, thinking or reading about the art of make-up will help you little. You must actually use make-up to acquire the knowledge and skill to enjoy it. When you do, you will find what little time it actually takes to really look your best.

Do some practicing by making up for the less important events of your everyday life. Don't put off learning what make-up is all about until a big event is a few hours away. You have neither the patience nor the free mood to acquire a new skill then. This leads only to frustration. Purchase the products you will need well in advance. Manufacturers are constantly improving old products and introducing new ones. Open them up at a quiet, leisurely moment at home. Examine them, experiment with them, become familiar with them. They will then pose no difficulties when you are ready to wear them.

The male is changing his feathers—not the mallard duck but the modern man, particularly the American. His clothing, for leisure as well as for business, has advanced steadily in fashionable cut, design and color. However, the real revolution is taking place in his grooming habits and his attention to personal appearance.

Cosmetics and Grooming Aids for the Male

Historically, with few exceptions, the male has contented himself with but a few basic and essential hygienic and grooming measures: skin cleansing (often limited in scope), beard shaving or shaping, and hair trimming and combing. Doing more than this could easily provoke comments from friends and associates. In the recent past the barber's conventional use of a pleasantly scented hair dressing was meekly tolerated; witch hazel and bay rum were excused as necessary "tonics" for freshly shaven skin. Most men eventually acquired such items as Father's Day or Christmas gifts. Home use of after-shave lotions, powders and hair preparations was irregular; the new year's gifts crowded out those received in previous years. The scope of products gets larger each year.

A man's skin suffers virtually the same aging processes as the woman's. With age his skin loses oil less rapidly than that of a woman. However, it reacts exactly as the woman's when exposed to sun, wind, cold, and dust. Many men have repeatedly borrowed their wives' hand cream, or face cream, particularly during the winter season, to relieve the discomfort of dry, chapped and irritated skin.

The male now has available to him many products designed and packaged to suit his needs, to keep his skin healthier, well cleansed and well fortified against the changes produced by environment and age. In addition to the established shaving and toiletry items, there are products available just to dress up the skin. All are male-oriented in appearance of the package and even in fragrance. No man should wait to receive them as a gift. Purchase them at local drugstores, special male "bars" in department and specialty shops as well as at haberdasheries that have traditionally catered to your wants.

The constant presence of such products will eventually result in experimentation—occasional use for a special event. When anticipated gibes from friends and associates just do not occur, more regular use becomes the pattern. Slowly comes the realization that manliness need not be compromised by the use of pleasantly scented after-shave lotions and talcs.

Fortunately, the message has gotten across that cleanliness and neatness can be considerably enhanced by antiperspirants, deodorants and even colognes. This message is now being forcefully delivered by sports heroes whose masculinity is unquestioned. Nevertheless, most of the male grooming aids still enter the home via gift package; only now they are being used—regularly, daily and unconsciously.

The sociologists will tell us why the mid-twentieth-century male was ready to accept this revolution in his habits. Whatever the reasons, however, it is here and spreading to all age groups and levels of society.

A balanced collection of men's products with a uniform fragrance throughout consists of:

1. Soap for cleansing face and hands.
2. Shampoo for scalp and/or the body.
3. A "pre-blade" beard softener to make shaving easier.
4. Shaving lather.
5. Two types of after-shave preparations:
   a. The standard lotion which is quite drying in its effects, stings as it enters tiny nicks and cuts, and is most suitable for the younger man with the oilier-type skin.
   b. A skin balm which lacks the bracing effect of the lotion and is particularly suited to the man whose skin is dry in texture. This product is best for the colder months and for the older man.
6. Hair-dressing products. In addition to the conventional grooming preparations, the hair may be kept in place with a hair spray. This permits a man with luxuriant scalp hair to maintain it neatly groomed in a "soft" manner, even outdoors.
7. Deodorant/antiperspirant creams, sticks and sprays.
8. Colognes.
9. A series of special products to promote better skin texture. A man's skin also loses oil as he gets older; usually his skin suffers more than a woman's from environmental exposure demanded by occupation and participation in outdoor sports.
   a. A skin-conditioning cream for face and hands particularly; adds moisture and oil to the skin to give it a smooth and comfortable feel. This is the type prod-

uct many men have used for years by raiding their wives' supply.

b. A cream for nighttime use which contains more oils. This is advantageous for the man who is experiencing excessively dry skin.

c. A mask-like product for improved skin cleansing without using soap. It is applied to the face, allowed to dry (usually in five to ten minutes) and then rinsed off.

10. Protective agents.

a. A sportsman's outdoor cream which not only lubricates the skin surface for wind and dust protection, but also shields the skin from the burning rays of the sun. Rubs in well and should be reapplied frequently. For use in all seasons.

b. Tanning gel for the man who is actively seeking sunlight and must acquire a good deep tan for self-satisfaction.

11. Products to improve appearance.

a. For years the five-o'clock shadow has been covered with flesh-tinted talcum powders. It has always done a poor job. It has now been improved. Cake powders in several shades are available. Not only is there a shade to match skin color, but the product now adheres to the skin to camouflage the beard and even out the skin tone. Applied with a special pad, the cake powder goes on the face without being showered over your clothing.

b. A face bronzer to impart an even, well-tanned appearance to your face in seconds. Available in several shades, it is non-permanent and can be washed off easily.

The above list is a rational collection of useful products specifically designed for men. If they seem to be duplicates of products used by women, it is only because the basic rules for skin hygiene are the same for both sexes.

The male has a basic, or inborn, timidity toward the use of cosmetics (and their purchase). I have found the skin bronzing cream an excellent convincer. It is easily and quickly applied to face, forehead, ears and neck. It dries quickly and blends to a healthy, sportsman's complexion tone that looks naturally acquired. In seconds your appearance is improved. It lasts for hours. By the time you wash it off at bedtime you will be convinced that cosmetics are for the male, too.

IX ADDING FRAGRANCE AND ELIMINATING ODOR

Perfume imparts a "fourth dimension" to people, places, and things.

Throughout this book my goal is to help you create or cultivate the most attractive physical image possible in business, at school, in social, or at leisure living. The emphasis is on the visual —how you look to friends, family and associates. However, the impression you create on those about you is a blend of several sensations. A sensation of singular importance is odor.

There are occasions when odor can contribute more than sight in establishing your presence. Odor can be recognized from any direction; it can skirt around corners. A direct line of vision is not necessary. It's startling how often an impressive odor will cause your head to turn to seek it out. Odor can be recognized even in the dark. Odor registers quickly, can be remembered and recalled; its appreciation is subject to education and adaptation. Do not minimize the influence of odor upon our patterns of behavior. The captains of industry learned long ago that merchandise can be sold by smell, whether it is the distinctive odor of a new car or the flavorful aroma of a package of chewing gum. The image you wish to create for yourself also depends upon fragrance.

Perfumery is a well-established and highly refined art. It has been a constant companion to man in every civilization. Odors have been used to protect from evil spirits and demons, to heal and cleanse the sick and to petition the gods. In the world of cosmetics and toiletries perfumery serves many functions. It disguises the usually unpleasant odor that results from the mixture of the necessary chemicals required to make a product. It also conveys distinctiveness and character as well as improved acceptability. The most important position of perfume rests with its ability to impart a pleasant, attractive odor upon your person in the creation and cultivation of the desirable, flattering image you wish to present to our demanding society.

A fragrance is an extremely complex mixture of the extract of natural substances such as flowers, leaves, roots, herbs, shrubs, animal exudates, and aromatic, synthetically produced, chemicals. All or part of these substances and chemicals are blended so as to yield a pleasing odor.

The perfume in the bottle can be a very different perfume when it is placed upon your skin. Once applied to the skin, the perfume is warmed by your body and gains "life." The odor it finally emits is influenced by the chemical substances that are distinctive to your skin: perspiration, natural skin oils and bacteria. This is why well-established brands of perfume yield odors that differ slightly from person to person. Of equal importance is the manner in which the fragrance dissipates itself; for like all living things it undergoes aging. A fine fragrance is one that is long-lasting; its odor will remain uniform as it slowly spends itself. You must give these factors careful consideration when you select a fragrance.

The professional perfumer classifies odors into many categories: floral, fruity, smoky, mossy, etc. These expressive names are of no practical value to you.

You use many scented substances simultaneously—hair spray, make-up, hand cream, etc. If such products have been properly designed, their odor will fade rapidly so as not to interfere with the fragrance which is produced by your main perfume. If your perfume has been designed properly, it will continue to emit its attractive fragrance, uniformly, for many hours.

PERFUME is the most concentrated and costly form in which a fragrance may be purchased. It contains fifteen to twenty per cent of its complex oil mixture in alcohol. A few small dabs upon the skin are all that is necessary to produce the emission of fragrance about your person.

A COLOGNE averages only about five to ten per cent oils in an alcohol-water combination; because it is diluted, its cost is not as great. Cologne must be used more liberally than a perfume. Large surface areas, such as your shoulders or arms, should be covered by the product.

An EAU DE TOILETTE is even more diluted and contains approximately five per cent oils in an alcohol-water diluent. For this reason it is usually applied freely to much of your body, as after the bath.

Obviously, the diluted fragrances do not have the staying quality of a perfume. Although in covering a large area the desired odor is emitted with strength, the increased skin surface activity promotes more rapid loss or decay of the fragrance.

Most manufacturers will produce their popular fragrances in at least two forms—the perfume and a cologne or eau de toilette. Although the odor of the diluted form is very similar to that of the perfume, it is not possible to make the two exactly the same. The complex perfume formula must be adjusted to withstand dilution. However, it takes an extremely educated nose to detect these subtle differences.

Remember that perfumes, colognes, or toilet waters require the warmth of your body and the opportunity to evaporate in order to work effectively. There seem to be many secret methods in some families on how and where it is best for putting on perfume. Practice whatever suits you best. In my opinion it is not how nor where but *what* you put on that is important.

I do know that there is no advantage in applying perfume to "pulse points"—areas of the skin, such as at the wrists, at which you can feel the pulsations of your heart. I also know that there is some advantage and also danger in saturating pieces of absorbent cotton with your favorite fragrance for insertion between your skin and undergarments at strategic locations. If the cotton is oversaturated and bulky, if there is too much pressure or friction between it and your skin and too little opportunity for evaporation, you can damage your skin.

A woman with a well-endowed bosom consulted me for second-degree chemical burns of her mid-chest which involved portions of both breasts. It was this lady's custom, on special occasions, to bury a cotton ball, saturated with perfume, in her bra between her breasts. On this occasion her bra may have been a bit too snug, or the cotton too moist, or the burial too deep! The alcohol of the perfume could not evaporate; pressure and friction over a period of hours produced a chemical burn of the skin which required two weeks to heal.

For convenience in application, fragrances are also available in pressurized aerosol devices and occasionally in stick form.

A dominant pleasing fragrance is a vital attribute to your grooming. Be a little inventive, a little adventurous; vary your perfume with mood, event, costume, time of day and season of the year.

The Control of Perspiration and Body Odor

In our modern society body odor must be eliminated. Fresh perspiration has no odor, although after some hours the bacteria that normally reside on your skin act upon perspiration. This *bacterial action yields a characteristic odor.* In addition, as mentioned in an early chapter on anatomy, there are special modified sweat glands concentrated in the armpits, about the nipples and genitals. The secretion of these glands is subject to much greater *bacterial action to produce a very typical odor.*

In the early stages of our evolutionary development, this characteristic apocrine scent may have played a significant role in sexual attraction. In our present-day society, normal body odor is considered offensive and wet armpits which stain clothing is embarrassing. Many products are available to help you satisfy the dictates of our society. They will be identified and discussed so that you may select the products that suit your individual needs.

Normal body temperature is maintained by

the evaporation of perspiration. Usually we are unaware this is happening; it is called insensible perspiration. When environmental temperature is high, as in the summer, or if you are in a very warm room, visible sweating takes place. Much of this perspiration, particularly in the presence of high humidity, will be absorbed by your clothing. Visible sweating can be provoked by factors other than heat. These are emotional tension, such as fear and anxiety; the ingestion of particular foods, such as spices and alcohol and medications; the presence of certain abnormal body states, as increased thyroid function.

The armpits are rich in both sweat and apocrine glands. Visible perspiration in this location may be annoying and embarrassing to you even if it is fresh and free of odor. Clothing becomes stained and uncomfortable. Although dress shields can be worn in the armpit area to absorb perspiration and protect clothing, these accessories are not suitable for all types of clothing and activities. They are clumsy to adjust and require particular laundering care. Although some women have learned to tolerate them, I have never known a man who could wear them.

The appearance of sweat on your skin surface can be reduced by the application of certain astringents. The most efficient and convenient are metallic salts such as aluminum chloride and sulfate. Dilute solutions of these substances, when applied to your skin, will actually reduce sweating for several hours. The degree of response will be better in some people than in others. However, in the vast majority of users, good sweat reduction takes place. The exact mechanism by which this occurs is not clearly understood and experts in the field are in disagreement.

Unfortunately, these salts, if not used carefully, can be irritating to skin. Upon becoming embedded in clothing they can be destructive to its fibers, particularly in the laundering and ironing process. However, the chemist has been able to modify these chemicals and prepare modern formulations that overcome these undesirable qualities. The following substances, alone or in combination, will reduce perspiration upon fresh application to the armpits. They can be found as *antiperspirants* at any toiletries counter: in creams for application via the fingers; lotions that may be applied by spray from a squeeze bottle, a pressurized aerosol or a "roll-on" applicator or similar dabbing device. Some of these have mild powers to destroy the skin bacteria that cause odor; therefore they are, to some degree, also deodorants:

aluminum chloride
aluminum chlorhydroxide
aluminum formate
aluminum sulfate
sodium aluminum lactate
zirconyl hydroxychloride

It is worth repeating that products which contain only the above substances, alone or in combination, are essentially antiperspirants. They will reduce the amount of perspiration delivered to the skin surface. They are only mild deodorants, since they have limited ability in counteracting the odor-forming bacteria of the skin. It is also true that with less perspiration on the skin, there is less for the skin bacteria to act upon to create an odor.

Deodorants are substances which influence

or alter body odor. This can be accomplished in either of two ways:

Directly, by applying acceptable fragrances to the body in sufficient strength to overcome or mask the odor considered undesirable. Perfumes, colognes and toilet waters function ideally to accomplish this.

Indirectly, by reducing the bacteria normally found on the skin surface so that bacterial decomposition of perspiration which is responsible for the undesirable odor is significantly reduced or prevented. No masking odor is added. You are merely avoiding the production of body odor. These products are primarily applied to the armpits where the concentration of perspiration and bacteria is very great. Their efficiency can be increased if the armpits are free of the hair which contributes to the entrapment of sweat and bacteria.

Deodorants are available at toiletries counters as: creams for application with the fingers; lotions for direct application via a roll-on device; sprays via a pressurized aerosol mechanism; bar or liquid soap products. Several commonly used active substances which perform in this manner are:

benzalkonium chloride
cetalkonium chloride
hexachlorophene
methylbenzethonium chloride
neomycin sulfate
parachlorometaxylenol
salicylanilides
thiuram disulfide
zinc phenolsulfonate

It must be remembered that these agents do not influence the production of perspiration; *they will not keep armpits dry.* They function exclusively to reduce odor. *Deodorants are not antiperspirants.*

Most people erroneously use these words as if they had the same meaning. Their composition and performance are very different. Failure to understand this may cause confusion and disappointment. You may be expecting a product to perform in a manner for which it was never designed.

Many manufacturers now make products that are both antiperspirants and deodorants. These contain combinations of ingredients from the two lists above; perspiration is diminished and bacterial action on perspiration is restricted to prevent or diminish the development of odor.

In selecting a product, consider your needs. A deodorant, for example, is of no use to you if you are disturbed by moist armpits. If you belong to the majority of Americans who prefer "complete coverage," then choose one of the combinations.

Many manufacturers market each type product in a variety of forms under a single brand name. However, a moment's consideration and a reading of the package label will permit you to select the kind of service you want in the precise form you find easiest to use.

Take an additional moment to read the directions for use on the package you purchase. Most of these products should not be applied to freshly shaved skin. Shaving removes some of the uppermost protective layer of the skin. In some individuals, tiny nicks or cuts may occur. The application of antiperspirants soon thereafter may cause skin irritation. With just a little planning you can shave your armpits before retiring in the evening. You will avoid difficulty on applying the antiperspirant the following day.

In the few instances of skin irritation of the armpits related to the use of antiperspirant-deodorant products which I have seen in private practice, the stories related to me have been quite uniform. Previous use of the product was without any difficulty. However, upon dressing for a special event one evening a dress other than that originally planned was selected. Suddenly this required cleanly shaved armpits, which seemed only a minor, hurried inconvenience. Since many women just don't feel properly dressed if their antiperspirant-deodorant is omitted, it was also applied to the freshly shaved areas. An immediate tingling sensation was experienced which developed into an uncomfortable irritation several hours later.

In discussion with each patient, I asked: "Don't you know you shouldn't use an antiperspirant-deodorant on broken skin with post-shaving nicks?"

The reply has been: "Yes, but I couldn't help it. I had no other dress to wear and it couldn't be worn without clean armpits."

"But then why did you use the antiperspirant-deodorant that very evening?" I asked.

"Oh, I couldn't go out without it on. I never do. And it seems to me I've put it on right after shaving before and never had any trouble."

It is, of course, possible to apply these products immediately after shaving without creating any problem, if care is taken to avoid nicking the skin. The manufacturer's directions should be followed. Fortunately, with a few days of medical supervision the skin eruption recovers completely and a lesson is learned the hard way.

There are no products available that completely control all excessive perspiration. If you perspire heavily, you can expect only modest reduction from the use of these externally applied preparations. Many complex internal factors may cause profuse perspiration over selected areas such as the hands and feet. This may become a serious, and at times almost disabling, complaint. Your physician can prescribe medication for internal use that can reduce the problem somewhat. Unfortunately, with adequate dosage these medications usually cause symptoms of their own that are as undesirable as the excessive perspiration.

Many encouraging studies are in progress, searching for answers to the more efficient control of excessive perspiration. From this effort will come new classes of compounds for either external application or internal use that will help this special group of patients.

PLASTIC SURGERY   X

Modern surgical skills can resculpture the face to correct scars, improve natural-born undesirable contours and hide the unflattering features that appear with the skin-aging process. However, the rules of the game are not the same as with conventional surgical procedures.

The face and neck—as indeed the entire body surface—are complex structures consisting of many planes and contours. The sculptured features they produce have a wide range of variation. However, for what we choose to call beautiful, handsome, or attractive, the limits of variation are restrictive. A prominently jutting jaw, jug handle ears, or a hooked nose are features that are outside such a conservative and wholly arbitrary limitation.

You, as an individual, create your own standards—what you like to see in others as well as what you would like to find in yourself. Life is a constant series of adjustments to these standards. This book is about the use of grooming aids and cosmetics that will help you bring about some of these adjustments. But, when the need for alteration is excessive—the removal of pouches about the eyes, the correction of a poor scar after an automobile accident —then surgical intervention is necessary.

I believe it is important that you understand how we "see" a scar, a wrinkled line, or a skin discoloration. Generally speaking, we prefer that surfaces, whether flat or curved, be smooth and even. Such a surface reflects light back to your eye uniformly. Your eye sees clear, unchanged light (see SKETCH 10–1a).

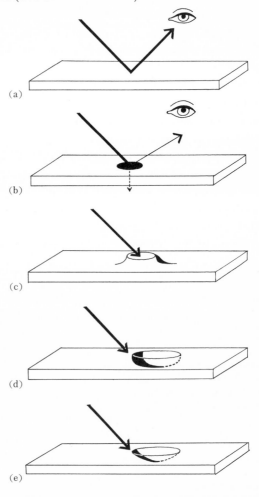

(a)

(b)

(c)

(d)

(e)

Depressions or elevations will specifically influence the lines of light that are reflected from such a surface. Shadows are produced that are directly related to the height of the elevation, the depth of the depression and other principal factors. These shadows are easy to "see"; they reveal the distortion of the surface (see SKETCHES 10–1c, d, e).

Waxing a table top or auto fender fills in and corrects minor defects, scratches, dust particles, etc. The polished surface becomes more pleasing because the light reflected from it to your eye reveals no shadows that the previous imperfections created.

A discoloration or a stain in a perfectly smooth surface absorbs some of the light that strikes that surface. The light reflected back to your eye is changed. You "see" the spot because its reflected light is different than that from the surface about it (see SKETCH 10–1b).

The influence of light and shadow on your skin is no different from that of the inanimate objects about you. The make-up you apply to your face corrects millions of tiny depressions, elevations, and discolorations in the skin to

SKETCH 10–1: *The distortions upon any surface— table top, car fender, or the living skin—are apparent to us by the manner in which light is reflected from them to our eye; or by the shadows the distortions create upon the surface. In (a) the surface is flawless— it reflects light directly back to the eye without any alteration. In (b) we "see" the black spot because the same light loses some of its intensity before it is reflected to the eye. The spot absorbs some of the light. In (c) we can observe an elevation in the surface because the light casts a shadow. In (d) the depression casts a shadow. Although the depression in (e) is as deep as in (d), it is less prominent because its wall is not as sharply defined—it has a gradual slope and casts a smaller shadow.*

permit its surface to reflect light uniformly. This achieves an attractive skin surface; it is more pleasing to the eye. Scars, pouches, wrinkle lines, birthmarks, moles, freckles, etc. therefore are noticeable because of the shadows they cast —the manner in which they reflect light in comparison to the surrounding skin. Modern plastic surgery corrects and improves these physical relationships.

Correction of Acquired Defects

Let us begin with a discussion of the revision or reduction of acquired defects—those which result from an injury or disease.

Suppose that an automobile accident has caused several lacerations about the head including the face. All the wounds heal promptly. The line of each scar is somewhat elevated. However, after several months nature itself is adequately and obviously correcting the problem. The skin surface is flattening out.

Unfortunately, one of the smallest of the wounds which had split the lip has healed with a puckering up of the red portion. The natural lip line is distorted. It is obviously not improving with time. While a full smile tends to even out the deformity, a half-smile may accentuate the defect. If this is the mouth of a girl, wearing lipstick adds to the problem.

The plastic surgeon has acquired special skills. He knows where and how to operate on this lip; what tissue, if any, should be removed; or from what cosmetically unimportant area new tissue may be taken to build up or fill in the old wound so that, upon healing, the least perceptible distortion remains.

The improvement he has accomplished is

readily apparent to all, including the patient. Although the final end result approaches, but cannot equal, that which preceded the accident, this physician, this mortal, has indeed wrought a minor miracle.

Satisfactory revision of such acquired defects, large and small, is an everyday occurrence. You should not allow an unattractive scar to affect your personality or earning capacity. Consult with a plastic surgeon as soon as possible.

Fairly common, non-life-threatening diseases have pronounced skin manifestations: simple infections, chicken pox, acne, several tropical or subtropical insect-borne diseases. Any of these skin conditions, on healing, may cause single or multiple scars. They may be as tiny as pin points or as large as coins. They are unattractive because they cause shadows and reflect light in a distorted manner. If this light distortion can be reduced, the shadows minimized, then improvement results. The plastic surgeon alone, or in concert with dermatologic colleagues, may utilize many techniques to achieve benefit by either simple removal (cutting out) of the entire defect, if isolated or few in number; or alteration of the architecture of the scars where many are present, as with multiple pock marks of the face.

A depression (scar) with sharp-angled walls distorts light more than a depression, equally as deep, but with gradually sloping walls (see Sketches 10–1d, e, p. 146). The skillful application of destructive chemicals, electric current or mechanical abrasion converts the individual sharp-walled scars to slightly larger but improved scars with sloping walls that cause less light distortion, less shadow casting. The methods are the same as that described under the treatment of warty growths and discolorations discussed in the chapter on aging skin.

Large surfaces of the skin are painted with a chemical which causes deep peeling (chemabrasion) of the skin. The procedure is somewhat painful and causes marked swelling of the tissues. While it sounds simple, the supervision of a physician is absolutely necessary; a period of from two to four days' hospitalization is required.

Virtually the same results can also be obtained by mechanical measures (dermabrasion). Large skin-surface areas are injected with an anaesthetic or frozen to board-like hardness by spraying with a special refrigerant. The skin is then scraped with wire brushes or burrs spinning at high speed. The upper layers of the skin are actually planed off. When the skin regenerates in eight to ten days the pock marks are less obvious because their former cup-like shape has been changed to a saucer-like shape with sloping walls that cast less shadow. The immediate healing period may be quite uncomfortable so that a two- to three-day hospital stay is desirable. The newly healed skin is pink compared to the untreated area; however, in a few weeks good blending occurs. With chemabrasion and dermabrasion, several treatments may be necessary to produce the results desired.

Isolated scars or even wrinkle lines may be treated with an electric current exactly like the one which is used to destroy superfluous hair. The fine needle is inserted into the wall of the deformity to destroy minute amounts of tissue; a deep-walled scar is converted to a shallow-walled defect which reflects light more pleasingly. This procedure is slow and tedious, causes little discomfort and is an office procedure.

From the foregoing, you can see that for many specific, acquired, obvious defects that may follow accident or disease, the skilled surgeon possesses many techniques which may be used alone, or in combination, to produce significant improvement in appearance—improvement that is obvious and welcome to all—patient, friends, etc.

There is another and equally important aspect of plastic surgery. This deals with changing the appearance of natural features: the shape of the nose or chin; the degree of protrusion of the ears; the removal of the bags about the eyes and/or jawline; the elimination of excess skin laxity in general; the correction of pronounced furrows as those about the mouth.

Alteration of Natural Features

The skilled surgeon can indeed modify these and many similar conditions. Such alterations are significant. Major contours and surface relationships of the face are being sculptured to present a different face.

At the crux of the endeavor is whether the change will conform to that which you have in mind. Will the new face match the mental image you have of yourself? If it does, you are satisfied. If it does not, there is disappointment; no matter how skillful and successful the surgery has been; no matter how pleasing your new features may appear to others.

Therefore, the plastic surgeon is interested in you as an individual: your personality and position in life; your work and ambitions; the motivation that brings you to him. He is interested in how you see yourself as well as how you think others see you. In short, do you have the stability and maturity to understand and accept the facial alteration that will be produced? If in the surgeon's judgment you do not, he will not accept you as a patient. And my friends doing plastic surgery tell me many individuals fall in this category. However, for the acceptable patient, the skills of the plastic surgeon will indeed result in great satisfaction and pleasure.

It is not feasible to describe the surgical procedure for the many correctible problems that exist. The principle is to remove excess tissue or to replace tissue where it is deficient; to produce flattering contours and smooth out surface areas; to hide incision lines behind ears, in the hairline, etc. so that the means by which the change was accomplished are not noticeable.

Unfortunately, *the improved status of a facelift operation for aging contours cannot be permanent;* nor can one predict for how long it will remain completely satisfactory, although the surgeon himself may, occasionally, make some estimation. You must not forget that the aging process continues. The face lift improves the aging contours that are present at the time of the surgery. The surgery cannot influence the aging effects that must naturally occur in the years that follow the procedure. Of course, some surgical procedures can be repeated to restore previous benefit.

The plastic surgeon himself, or one of his trained assistants, is eager and anxious to discuss every phase of the surgery program with you: the procedure itself, the duration of hospitalization, discomfort, length of disability, after-care, etc. In addition, you will be advised of the fee which may range from $100 for a simple, single office procedure to several thousand dollars for detailed and extensive work. Since most medical insurance policies do not provide benefits for this type of elective surgery, you must be fully aware of this important detail. Do not be surprised if you are required to pay the entire fee in advance. This is quite standard procedure and completely ethical for this special form of surgery.

Much has been written in the popular press in recent years about silicone injections. It has created much interest and deserves mention in this chapter.

Silicone is a synthetic, rather thick, heavy, oil-like, clear fluid which can be injected into tissue by a standard hypodermic syringe and needle. Unlike paraffin-type substances that have been tried in the past, silicone appears to have several important and attractive advantages upon tissue instillation.

The injection procedure is simple and quite painless; following insertion it permits external manipulation so that the operator can actually mold the material to some degree to conform to normal-type skin-surface contours. Most important of all, the silicone seems not to promote any inflammatory reaction in the surrounding tissue and tends to remain in the area of the immediate site of injection without wandering. The skin texture and "feel" appear normal.

Obviously, such a material and simple procedure seem ideal for correcting defects caused by an absence of tissue, such as: depressed scars, furrows, wrinkle lines, or even the extensive problems of the non-symmetrical face with which some children are born. Much publicity has been given to its use in building up breasts.

At the time of this writing, the substance and the procedure have been the subject of careful investigation by a mere handful of physicians in several medical centers about the country. These have been the only doctors authorized by the Food and Drug Administration to administer and study the benefits, and any possible dangers, that may take place from silicone injections. The results appear very promising. There is no doubt that the work will not only continue but probably expand in scope. As knowledge is gained, it is possible that, in the near future, more physicians will be authorized to join the program.

However, silicone injections are not generally available in the U.S.A. and will not be for several more years.

THE GLORY OF HAIR XI

Some prefer it waved, others want it straight. Some like it blonde while some prefer it brunette. Some have too much, while others complain they have too little; yet others are distressed because they have hair in the wrong place completely! A wealth of products, procedures and devices offers help to everyone— male and female.

Hair and its appearance have played significant roles in man's culture, religion, society and politics. Boys in ancient Greece, upon attaining manhood, would cut their hair and dedicate it to the gods. In the middle ages short hair, even among men, was the mark of a slave; but by the fifteenth century, as armor was worn, short hair became a necessity. Women's hair fashions also went through many phases: from being decorously covered to being fantastic creations draped over wire foundations and adorned with jewels, feathers, even baskets of fruit. The use of wigs and false hair was popular at various times in both French and English society; these customs were also brought to the New World.

In our twentieth century, hair styles continue as important forms of expression. Aroused

Europeans, as the war ended in 1945, sheared off the hair of women who collaborated with the enemy. Today some of our young people are growing long hair as a form of protest.

Three particular events in our century have had a profound effect on hair fashions: a new freedom to styling began with the popularization of bobbed hair by the dancer Irene Castle; a method of permanent waving was introduced by Charles Nessler; and simple, safe, color alteration was achieved by modern advances in bleaching and tinting. Hair coloring, mainly to hide grey hair, dates back to about 400 B.C. However, the ability to achieve and maintain a particular and attractive color shade is only a recent accomplishment.

In personal grooming your hair exerts tremendous influence on the appearance you create. It emphasizes your face as a frame to a picture, but more so. Hair shapes not only your head but your entire body by influencing your neck, shoulders and even your height. Your coiffure, your make-up and your costume must complement each other to create the attractive image you want to project.

Hair may be the object of special attraction, and consequently it may be an important factor in the relationship between a man and a woman. Some wives have learned that changing hair length or color is a means for improving domestic bliss.

In an earlier chapter we discussed some of the characteristics of scalp hair growth and structure. The hair filament itself, for simplicity's sake, can be considered as a strand of protein with an inner core; the medulla, surrounded by an outer core; the cortex, which contains the pigment to give the hair its natural color. The outermost surface is hard and shiny and is called the cuticle. In the normal or virginal hair, the protein molecules are carefully joined together to give the hair shaft a smooth, strong surface that has a pleasant silky texture. The sheen is produced by the uniform reflection of light characteristic for a sleek surface. That is why the still surface of a pond looks so shiny. When a surface is rough—a rippled pond, for instance—light is reflected in a haphazard and dull fashion.

The texture and gloss of your hair is also influenced by a thin coating of natural oil from the scalp glands. In time, however, the accumulation of oil becomes dull as it is oxidized by air. The deposition of dust and soil add surface tarnish and weight to each shaft. Your hair must be washed to restore its sheen and usual spring.

Dandruff

The scalp is subject to a particularly common hygienic problem—*dandruff*—that may influence your personal comfort as well as the grooming and appearance of your hair. Oddly enough, the precise cause of this ancient disorder has not been established. Although bacteria and related elements are found in association with this scalp condition, there is no conclusive evidence that dandruff is caused by any microorganism. It is not contagious!

There is a definite relationship between dandruff and the well-developed oil glands of the scalp. Often the disorder is especially troublesome during the acne period and early adulthood. However, no age group is spared and men and women are equally affected.

Flaking and itching of the scalp itself are the principle features of dandruff. Flakes can also be seen directly on the hair or showered over dark clothing to convey a very unkempt appearance. The scurf may become pronounced and persistent with episodes of aggravated symptoms in the late spring and fall; occasionally erosions (open areas) of the scalp may appear. Because of internal body influences, external treatment may improve or control the manifestations of dandruff without establishing a long-lasting cure.

Conventional shampoos, hairdressings, and "tonics" offer limited benefit in the management of dandruff since they merely free and/or rinse away loose scales which quickly reform. More effective care requires the application of preparations containing agents similar to that used in the treatment of acne (sulfur, salicylic acid, resorcinol, parachlorometaxylenol, tars, etc.) or special items such as selenium sulfide or corticosteroids which your physician must prescribe.

Often effective "anti-dandruff" remedies are inelegant, troublesome, time-consuming or not conducive to regular and persistent use. A new compound has recently been developed that helps control even severe dandruff problems. Its chemical name is *zinc pyrithione*, and it is presently available in a greaseless cream hairdressing or a shampoo. Both convenient and pleasant products, particularly the hairdressing which remains on the scalp and on the hair between shampoos, encourage regular and repeated use to keep dandruff under control indefinitely.

The Shampoo For hair that has never been bleached, tinted, or waved, select a shampoo depending upon whether your scalp deposits little, average or much oil between washings. These are known as dry, normal or oily hair shampoos. Almost all modern shampoos are detergent mixtures rather than soap alone; they offer important advantages. Unlike soap, detergents are not affected by the hardness (amount of mineral components) of water. Soap does react with these minerals in water to form insoluble "salts," some of which (like the ring around a bathtub) are deposited on the hair shafts and reduce sheen. Detergents do not form such salts. In addition, the oil-removing capacity of detergents can be conveniently regulated. This permits the manufacture of the three types of shampoos mentioned.

Apply the shampoo to your wet hair and scalp; work it into the scalp by finger (not hand) massage. The fingers will reach to the scalp surface through the blanket of hair to loosen scurf (normal skin shedding), oil and soil. Then you can draw out the lather along the full length of your hair. If your hair is long, divide your scalp into four quarters. Then draw the lather, in turn, through each quarter section of hair. Finally, bring the four quarters together into a single full coil. This will reduce tangle and make the later combing process much easier. Rinse with copious amounts of clear water that are allowed to flow through your hair. A spray nozzle that can be held close to the scalp and hair does the best job. The nozzle should be attached to the water source by a flexible tube so that it can be freely moved about your head. Do not let the water strike your scalp and hair with great force. This strains and scatters the hair, adding unnecessary tension and tangle. For greater efficiency, give yourself two short shampoos and rinses rather than one long one.

Allow the excess water to drain off. Then

carefully wrap your hair in a soft absorbent towel. You may gently press the towel against the hair. *Do not rub.* This is particularly important to men and women who are noticing an increase in hair loss. *Rubbing with a towel multiplies the area of friction to produce tremendous damaging tension on the hair shafts.* The mechanical advantage that makes it easier to twist off a stubborn pickle jar cover by grasping it with a towel, also works to loosen and break off hair.

Some people like to check for cleanliness at this point by listening for a "squeak" when the hair is rubbed between the fingers. This is true; but the squeak also means that a little too much natural oil has been removed from the hair shaft.

If it is not convenient for you to allow your hair to dry spontaneously, use any one of the many circulating, warmed-air machines to speed up the process.

Hair that has been tinted and bleached, waved or straightened has an altered surface structure. The hard outermost coating (cuticle) has minuscule splits in it. These are too tiny to be seen with the naked eye, but they are sufficient to change the feel of the hair. It is less soft, less flexible and, because it reflects light differently, has less sheen. Special shampoo formulas have been developed for such hair. First, they will be most protective of the coloring which has been added to the hair; second, they are of a weakly acid nature rather than alkaline. This acidity temporarily closes up the little splits in the cuticle to make the tinted and bleached hair less porous than usual. Each hair shaft will then absorb less water when it is wet, thereby making it easier to manage. Otherwise the washing procedure is the same as for virginal hair, although somewhat more care should be taken to prevent tangling.

Special rinse rituals have been a part of folklore handed down for generations. There is considerable merit to some of them. This may account for the number of loyal followers each has.

Probably the most popular rinse is to add a small quantity of vinegar or lemon juice to the rinse water to give the hair more luster. Actually this is a weak, acid rinse; it reduces the film of hard water salts that soaps allow to be deposited on the hair shafts. However, the modern popular detergent shampoos work equally well in hard or soft water and dulling films are no longer a problem.

The second type of home-style rinse is to use beer or beaten egg in diluted forms to give the hair body. The sugar and protein from such rinses are deposited on the hair shafts to add weight, stiffness and some considerable stickiness.

Well-formulated commercial rinses are available to produce better and more uniform results with ease and cosmetic elegance, free of the earthy smells of the bar or kitchen.

A standard commercial *cream rinse* is formulated to promote sheen, neutralize the static charge of electricity that often follows hair washing, and increase the "slip" of the hair to make combing much easier. Apply to the wet hair and then gently flush out with clear water.

If you wish to impart weight and body to your hair (this is particularly for the beer and egg proponents), rinse your damp hair with a *set-*

ting lotion; do not flush out with water. This will remove (neutralize) any static charge of electricity, and coat the hair with a non-tacky transparent film that will stiffen it slightly for ease in combing and styling.

Whether you have virginal or tinted and bleached hair, use either or both of the above products to suit your own needs. However, with repeated tinting, bleaching and waving procedures, the hair shafts acquire greater architectural alteration of the cuticle and cortex. As more and more splits and cracks occur in the cuticle, the substance of the hair becomes more porous. Such hair requires special attention. A mild, detergent shampoo designed for such hair should be used followed by a cream rinse. Added benefit will accompany the use of a *hair conditioner.* These are cream preparations that are applied to the entire length of the hair by gently pulling the strands of hair through your cream-coated fingers. It is followed by a water rinse. Such conditioners tend to fill up the splits in the hair cuticle to give added strength. While this does not produce permanent restoration, it does prepare such hair to better withstand the setting, combing and styling procedures that follow.

A dry shampoo has recently found some favor. This is an adsorbent powder, such as a high grade talc, which permits soil, oil and grime to adhere to its particles. The powder is dusted over and into the hair, or even sprayed on from an aerosol can. After a few moments the hair must be toweled and brushed to remove the powder with its adherent soil.

Such shampooing has a few advantages. The hair can be cleansed quickly with a minimum of effort. Since it is not made wet, there is only little alteration in the hair set. Where wetting and drying the hair poses a health hazard, as with children, the dry shampoo has been helpful. Unfortunately, the scalp and hair do not get as clean as with a detergent shampoo. The brushing that is required increases the charge of static electricity, making manageability difficult.

Occasionally, despite the shampoo you use or the cream rinse you apply, static electricity can pose a problem in dry climates or in winter when indoor humidity is very low. With each brushing and combing the electric charge increases. Wetting the comb or brush, or the hair itself, will reduce this unmanageability. If greater control is required, a little oil is a better electrical insulator than water. Just place a few drops of a scented bath oil on your comb or brush. Men will prefer to use a hairdressing to manage their hair and give it an attractive sheen.

Setting and Styling

Setting, combing, and styling hair is an art that is the slave of fashion. Within the scope of this book, it is only possible to discuss the mechanics involved and the actual physical effects upon the hair itself.

Hair is almost entirely protein. It absorbs small amounts of water. If, however, the cuticle (outermost surface) has splits in it, such as results from tinting, bleaching and waving, the hair becomes porous. It will imbibe much more water than in the virginal state. Wet hair, when placed in a curled or rolled position, will tend to temporarily hold that shape to some degree when it dries. This is a common characteristic of all natural fibers. Wool, which is chemically closely related to hair, demonstrates this well. If you sit down in a wool garment wet from the rain, you know how easily it wrinkles. This is the very principle at work when hair is placed on rollers. The more porous the hair, the more water it absorbs, the better the hold of the wave. Virginal hair, therefore, is more difficult to set—children's hair particularly.

Placing the hair on rollers or pinning it in curled positions does not damage the hair shaft itself. However, under certain conditions, it is possible to weaken the hair filament at its attachment, in the follicle below the surface of the skin. Persistent pulling or tension of the hair at its attachment, over long periods of time, such as overnight, can do this.

To reduce this possible injury: Be sure to allow considerable "play" between the scalp surface and the pinned roller. You should always be able to lift the pinned roller away from your scalp easily and freely. As the completed pinned roller hangs in place, it must not be so heavy as to exert undue pull on the hair. The lightweight, small rollers are preferred. Many small rollers exert less tension than fewer heavier ones. A cap or kerchief will help to keep the rollers in place and reduce tension. Rollers or pinned curls should remain in place for short periods of time only. Sleeping in them as a regular or frequent procedure is unwise. Change your hair style frequently to allow sections of the scalp to rest from rolling and curling.

An important warning: If you use bobby pins, do not open them with your teeth. They can be conveniently opened with one hand by pushing the pin against the edge of a wedge-shaped piece of metal or plastic. You can easily purchase or make such a wedge for your dressing table. I have often been distressed to see patients with a worn-down front tooth. They were unaware that opening pins with the teeth was causing damage to their smile.

Although combing and brushing the hair is a simple routine, you must be aware of a few basic principles. Select a comb that will not bend easily under pressure. Its teeth should be uniformly spaced throughout the width of the comb and be of medium density; teeth that are too closely placed (the fine comb) can exert excessive friction on the hair shaft. Brushes should be of natural bristle, rather than synthetic-type fiber. Their stiffness should be sufficient to accomplish the dressing purpose for which they are designed. Natural bristles have rounded ends; synthetic fibers usually have sharply squared ends that may actually increase the wear upon your hair.

When stroking with your brush or comb, make long gentle passes through your hair. Don't snap the comb at the edge of the stroke. If there is a tangle, concentrate on that area to separate the shafts with fingers or comb. Don't include it in the next pass with a lot of neighboring hair. If the tangle persists, be sure to hold the hair closest to the scalp with your free hand as you try to free the tangle with the comb in the other hand. This will reduce tension on the hair at its attachment to the scalp.

Hair should be combed and brushed just long enough to make it look neat or to achieve the shape and style you want. Beyond that, excessive wear and damage will take place. "Split ends" are a sign of such damage. To my knowledge, there has never been a scientific study that revealed any advantage to brushing the hair one hundred strokes daily. It may possibly add some sheen, but the disadvantages to the ritual are real, especially for hair that has been tinted, bleached or waved. Unnecessary manipulation of any kind to such hair will only add to the risk of breaking the shafts. Remember, the hair filament is not a living structure. While it does replace itself, the hair you see and work with will wear like any fur. Would you brush your fur coat one hundred strokes each night?

Teasing or back-combing is a technique to achieve "body" or structuring of the hair mass; this is necessary for the bouffant or sculptured coiffures. A lock of hair is held away from the head; with many short, quick strokes with a fine comb, the hair is "combed" in the reverse direction—towards the scalp. This roughens the hair shaft by lifting up tiny sections of the hair's outer coating (cuticle). The hair shafts snag with their neighbors just as a nylon stocking snags to rough skin. By systematically repeating this procedure, it is possible to build the hair upon itself to achieve special styling effects.

Since the cuticle of the virginal hair shaft is intact and very hard, teasing or back-combing such hair is usually not very successful. Tinted, bleached or waved hair, with many splits in its surface, teases easily. Combs with teeth of uneven length have been designed to improve the efficiency of the teasing procedure. Aside from the fact that this, as any, added manipulative procedure may increase hair breakage, there is no harm to the actual growing capacity of the hair itself.

The Hair Spray   When your hair has been carefully combed and coaxed into the desired shape and position, you can easily maintain it so for hours by covering it with an invisible hair spray.

Hair sprays contain, basically, a film-forming plastic ingredient. In years past this was a shellac. In all modern products this film-former is now a synthetic compound, packed in an aerosol can. Upon activating the button of the can, a spray of fine droplets is produced to deposit an invisible film upon the hair. This coating will keep the coiffure together by diminishing the displacement that results from general activity. It will even resist the effects of wind and moisture.

Any type of hair style—the bouffant, sculptured or casual—will wear better and longer if it has been sprayed. Less effort and time is required to maintain a freshly groomed appearance. Most important, it spares fragile hair from additional manipulation.

Hair sprays vary in formula and differ in quality. Their performance will depend essentially upon the type and amount of film-forming ingredients they contain. Select a hair spray with thought. Consider the texture and styling of your hair; the amount and degree of exposure to which it is subjected. The film formed by the spray must be invisible and protective, but also free of tackiness, lest it attract dust particles. Hair spray fragrance should be pleasant, but never lingering lest it overpower your personal perfume.

When applying the spray, hold the can about ten inches from your hair. This is the best distance for achieving maximum deposition of the product in the most uniform manner. At too close range, many of the droplets will bounce off your hair and not be deposited at all. At a distance that is too great, many droplets may not reach your hair. Move the spray to get the best coverage; take care to avoid the eyes. It is a good practice to shield the eyes with your free hand when you spray the front of your head. For reasons of personal comfort do not inhale the spray. Reliable scientific studies have confirmed that there is no hazard to the lungs on repeated inhalation of hair sprays.

Hair Coloring In the past decade, hair coloring has entered a remarkable era. The concept has gained general acceptance by both men and women. Recent technical advances achieved by hair and cosmetic chemists are responsible for the impetus of this revolution. They have accomplished an ease and safety of application plus an expansive selection of permanent colors that was not previously dreamed possible.

This discussion will include the old as well as the new, the professional as well as the home-oriented products for coloring hair. There are many. Each performs in a particular manner. Select the one which best satisfies your needs.

To bring this topic into focus, I will begin with the important steps necessary before coloring hair. Remember that hair coloring is a skill. The very best results are obtained by experienced "hair colorists" in salons. However, it is possible for you to achieve complete satisfaction with the several products particularly designed for home use provided you follow meticulously all the directions supplied with each product.

The Patch Test Let us first consider a most important safety measure, absolutely required for users of most hair coloring processes. It is the skin patch test.

In the chapter on allergy, you learned that every substance has the potential for sensitizing the skin to cause it to break out in a rash. Fortunately, this potential to sensitize the skin is very low for substances used in cosmetics, and individuals who will develop an allergic rash are extremely rare in our population.

A few hair dyes and dye components formed at the time the chemical reactions take place to impart color to the hair have a higher potential to sensitize the skin than the usual cosmetic preparation. These dye substances belong to a family of chemicals commonly used to dye furs and fabrics; consequently anyone has an adequate opportunity to develop a skin sensitivity (allergy) to these chemicals before ever being exposed to a hair coloring product.

Just as was illustrated with the example of poison ivy, prior exposure to the allergy-producing substance is absolutely necessary to create an allergic state. This allergic state, when it occurs, does so in few individuals; it need not occur ever at all despite repeated exposure to the substance. For reasons unknown, an allergy may develop only after there have been many, many previous exposures.

Consequently, it is very important to determine that your skin is free of allergy to the hair dye product before you use it to color your hair. The test for this is a simple one. It requires no unusual knowledge, skill or experience to be interpreted properly. Originally, it was customary for salon colorists to select for the test a portion of skin behind their patron's ear; often, but not necessarily, the test area would include the hairline nearby. Such a location, however, cannot be viewed by a person who wants to color his own hair with a product designed for home use. Therefore, another and far more accessible skin site is recommended. It is the area of skin in front of the elbow, that portion which folds in as the elbow is flexed and stretches out for convenient viewing when the elbow is straightened. Since this skin is soft, thin, and easy to see, it makes an excellent test site.

The test procedure begins twenty-four hours before the hair is to be colored. Gently cleanse the test site, about 1½ inches in diameter, with mild soap, rinse with warm water and pat dry. In a vial or glass, mix a small amount of the toning lotion bottle with an equal amount from the color developer or peroxide bottle. These are the bottles that eventually will be mixed together to make the lotion for application to your hair. Using a cotton-tipped applicator apply (see SKETCH 11–1) the freshly mixed test material from the vial or glass to the prepared skin in front of your elbow. Leave it uncovered and in place for *twenty-four hours.* You must be care-

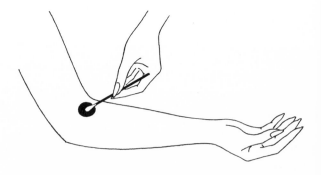

SKETCH 11–1: *The skin patch test: With a cotton-tipped applicator apply the freshly mixed test material to a previously cleansed area of skin in the bend of the elbow. Allow it to remain in place, uncovered, for at least 24 hours.*

ful not to rub or wash off the test substance during that time to assure a valid test. Long experience has shown that this time interval, for this thin skin site and concentration of the test material, is adequate to reveal the presence of skin allergy.

At the end of the twenty-four-hour period, gently cleanse the test site with clear warm water. Observe it. If the skin is red, irritated, bumpy or itchy, then it reveals that you may be allergic to the hair coloring preparation. *It must not be used by you.* If the test site is free of any skin reaction, then you may proceed to color your hair according to the directions provided by the manufacturer.

This is the patch test. There is no shortcut to it. It cannot be avoided. Since it is possible that your skin may become allergic to the hair coloring preparation during the weeks between uses, it is necessary that the test be repeated for the full twenty-four-hour period before each hair coloring session. This simple test is but a small inconvenience to assure safety and satisfaction in the fascinating process of achieving an attractive and permanent change in hair color.

Governmental regulation does not permit the use of these preparations to dye the eyebrows or eyelashes. The origin of this restriction is many years old, before patch tests were recommended, and at a time when highly purified raw materials were not readily available for manufacturing hair color products. The region of the eye presents distinct problems in application and possibilities for injury. Further discussion of this rigid and specific regulation is not within the scope of this book.

The Strand Test Hair, like fabric, may accept color in an unexpected manner. This is especially true if previous color has been applied to your hair. Since some methods for coloring hair are permanent —will not wash out—it is imperative that the manufacturer's instructions be carefully read and completely understood before you make any attempt to color your hair.

It is a simple matter to tie off a few dozen of your hairs with a length of strong sewing thread; cut this hair strand as close to the scalp as possible. Now examine the strand in your hand under a good light, daylight if possible. If color had been applied to your hair some weeks previously, you can easily compare it with your natural color in the new hair growth.

Since you already prepared a little of the hair coloring product for the patch test, you can use the same fresh material to color the strand to see how your hair will accept the color you intend to use. Follow the label instructions completely. Leave the material on the strand for the full time recommended by the manufacturer before rinsing it out. Re-examine the strand under the same good light, daylight preferred. Then believe what you see on the treated strand of your hair. That is exactly what is going to happen when the product is applied to the hair on your head.

If your hair was previously colored with chemicals not compatible with the product you intend to use, the manufacturer's directions with the package will instruct you exactly how to pretreat your hair before performing the strand test and before applying the product. If you are not satisfied with the results obtained in the strand test, or if you do not understand the package label and instructions, *then you must not proceed with coloring your hair.* Take your problem to a professional—your local beauty salon hair-colorist.

Going Lighter

To lighten your hair by more than one or two shades, or to achieve special light color effects, first remove all or much of the color that is present, whether it is your own or was artificially applied. This bleaching process is called "stripping" the hair. When thoroughly stripped, the hair has yellowish, straw-like color.

Bleaching chemicals are strong oxidizing agents of which the best known is twenty volume (6 percent) hydrogen peroxide. The bleaching mixture must be freshly prepared. An activating powder or liquid is added to the peroxide. For ease of handling and maximum efficiency, commercial bleaches have a creamy lotion consistency. They cling well to the hair while keeping contact with the skin to a minimum. This is most desirable, for the stronger peroxides may be irritating to skin. Very rarely do they cause an allergic reaction. Only an expert is qualified to test for it.

Upon contact with the skin, a very few individuals may experience a warming, tingling and sometimes painful sensation after several minutes. Although alarming at first, the experienced individual quickly acquires a tolerance to the discomfort. Should the distress become extreme, the bleach must be rinsed out immediately. Further stripping procedures are not recommended.

It may take as long as an hour or even more to satisfactorily strip your hair. The length of time depends upon the depth of color present as well as the thickness and texture of your hair. A plastic cap placed over the bleach-covered hair or exposure to heating lamps may improve the efficiency of the chemicals and help to reduce the time required for the process to reach completion. The heating lamps require special skills. They are not recommended for home use.

The basic components of bleaches are essentially the same; however, some manufacturers have formulated products which cause little to no discomfort while maintaining superior bleaching ability. If skin discomfort is a problem to you, it is worth switching brands. Some slight redness to your scalp may occasionally be noticed after a stripping procedure. If the redness is pronounced or discomfort great, it is best not to attempt coloring your hair the same day. If, with each future stripping procedure, your discomfort increases, ask your salon operator to change the product. If this does not meet with success, it is prudent to abandon the method entirely. Very few individuals have found this necessary.

When the hair has been stripped satisfactorily, the bleach is rinsed out and the yellow-orange hair is now ready to be colored to the light shade you have selected. The procedure for applying the toner (coloring mixture) is exactly the same as described below for the organic, oxidation-type permanent colors.

The Touch Up After six to eight weeks your new hair growth, which everyone incorrectly calls "the roots," appears obvious. This occurs because your hair was toned to a shade much lighter than your normal hair color. If you wish to maintain the same or a similar light shade, it is necessary to bleach this new growth. The bleaching agent is applied to the new growth only (unless a significantly different final color is to be applied to your hair). Your bleached "roots" and the remainder of your hair are now ready for toning in the usual manner.

Repeated bleaching and toning will cause more and more alteration to the cuticle of each hair shaft. Your hair may become brittle with a straw-like feel. It will be less able to withstand manipulation. Care will be required to avoid breakage. You can improve the appearance and feel of such hair by the frequent use of a hair conditioner.

When "roots" are being bleached during a touch-up, be sure to protect the remainder of the hair with a conditioner. In addition, your hair should receive regular applications of conditioner in the weeks between touch-ups. For details refer to the previous section on shampooing tinted and bleached hair. Let me emphasize that repeated bleaching and toning, regardless of frequency, *does not alter or diminish the natural growth ability of your hair*. Your new hair growth proceeds in normal fashion, constantly replacing hair that is clipped off or broken off. For this reason, it is possible at suitable intervals to indefinitely repeat the process of bleaching and toning the hair to desired shade.

1. THE ORGANIC, OXIDATION-TYPE DYE PRODUCT is by far the best method for coloring hair. You can recognize it by its two separate components: (1) a color, dye, or toner and (2) a developer (a chemical, like hydrogen peroxide which gives off the oxygen required for the chemical reaction). These must be mixed together just before use to form a lotion for im-

Types of Hair Coloring Agents

mediate application, with gloved hands, directly to the hair. It is left in place for approximately thirty minutes, then rinsed out. The hair is ready to be set, dried, combed out, and styled as desired. A skin patch test is required as discussed in detail previously. Once mixed, the product must be used immediately or discarded.

Advantages: It is permanent. The dye, in the presence of oxygen, enters the inner portion (cortex) of the hair shaft, becomes insoluble and will not wash out with subsequent shampoos. It is available in a broad spectrum of colors with the most natural tones. It will also provide the best coverage of grey with excellent color depth to blend with your natural hair. You may, if you wish, actually achieve a color that is several shades lighter or darker than your natural hair color with this single application. This method does not conflict with future permanent waving or hair straightening procedures. If, in the future, you should desire a significant change in color, you may bleach it out with ease.

Disadvantages: Summer sun and excessive perspiration may eventually cause some fading of the darker color components so that a reddish tone may be evident. After six to eight weeks, as new hair growth occurs, the coloring procedure may be repeated in order to maintain uniformity in appearance. The progressive use of this product will cover the new hair growth while maintaining an even and attractive tone elsewhere.

2. A NON-PEROXIDE, NON-OXIDATION, ORGANIC DYE PRODUCT is available to color hair. You can recognize this type product by its heavy lotion consistency, offered in a single package unit.

There is nothing to mix. Most manufacturers of such products provide sufficient lotion for two complete applications. After the first use, simply recap and store for the two to four weeks between applications. A skin patch test before each use is usually required. Unlike the oxidation-type dye discussed first, which actually penetrates to the cortex of the hair shaft, this non-oxidation product binds itself to the exterior (cuticle) of the hair only. The directions usually recommend that the lotion remain on the hair for approximately thirty to forty-five minutes before it is rinsed out.

Advantages: The color is reasonably good through three or four shampoos. It provides particularly adequate coverage for grey hair.

Disadvantages: The range of colors available is not wide. This product permits you to depart from your normal hair color only to a very limited degree, and then only to a shade that is darker than your own. You may notice some temporary skin staining after this type dye is rinsed from your hair. Sunlight, excessive perspiration, permanent waving, or straightening will all change the color. Repeated use eventually produces "build-up"—color on color—to impart a rather unnatural dark appearance to your hair. This color is not removed easily with decolorizer; the stained shafts make future use of an oxidation-type dye (#1 above) more difficult.

3. A NON-PEROXIDE, NON-OXIDATION, METAL-COMPLEXED, ORGANIC DYE is also available. It is a thick lotion, packaged in a single unit. There is no mixing. However, you can distinguish it from #2 since the package usually contains sufficient material for about four separate applications. A skin patch-test before each

use is usually required. This preparation also binds itself to the exterior cuticle of the hair rather than penetrating it. The usual directions suggest that it remain on the hair for ten to twenty minutes before being rinsed out.

Advantages: The color remains reasonably fast through four or more shampoos. If you have naturally grey, smoky, silvery or platinum-colored hair, you will find this product provides good coverage. It also blends well to cover the yellowing and to tone down the brassiness that is occasionally found in naturally light or grey-colored hair. Unlike #2 above, it is reasonably color-fast to sunlight and excessive perspiration. It is also more resistant to color alteration following permanent waving or hair straightening.

Disadvantages: The range of colors is very limited. You can only use shades that are darker than your own, but not very much so. Although the grey shades cause negligible skin staining, the darker shades may produce significant skin staining. That is why dark shades are not readily available in this type product. As with product #2, repeated use will produce "build-up" and darkening, but to a much lesser degree. This color is also not easily removed so that if you intend to use an oxidation-type dye in the near future, you will experience some difficulty.

4. NON-PEROXIDE, NON-OXIDATION, ORGANIC DYES IN ALCOHOL AND WATER SOLUTIONS are another hair-coloring-type product. Essentially, they are dilute solutions of dyes similar to products #2 and #3. You will find them as single bottles, usually with a flip-top squirt spout, containing eight to ten complete applications. A skin patch test before each use is usually required. The solution is applied to the hair and left in place. It is not rinsed out. Sometimes

color products of this type are incorporated with setting or grooming lotions.

Advantages: These are available in a broad spectrum of colors.

Disadvantages: A very limited change from your normal hair color is possible, and then only to a darker shade. Products of this type do not cover grey well, although they do blend grey down to make it less noticeable. It will usually last through only one or two shampoos. The color may actually rub off onto bed clothing; it is not very resistant to rain water. The residual staining of the hair that occurs can interfere with future coloring procedures.

5. CERTIFIED ORGANIC DYES. A certified dye is one that has been particularly designated by the U. S. Food and Drug Administration for use in foods, drugs and cosmetics. This product is packaged in a multi-application bottle. No skin patch test is required; however, it does bear the usual warning against use about the eyes. The lotion is applied to the hair and left in place. Do not rinse since it is easily washed out.

Advantages: This type of color product produces no residual staining to complicate future use of other hair color procedures. Very little rub-off to bed clothing occurs and there is good resistance to rain water.

Disadvantages: It is only possible to darken hair with products of this type. Its ability to cover grey is only modest. Some fading occurs on exposure to sunlight.

6. SIMPLE ORGANIC DYES are packaged in multi-application units: as powders in packets or capsules, in liquid or cream form in bottles or tubes. A dye solution is made by adding a measured amount of powder, liquid or cream to water. This solution is repeatedly rinsed through

the hair. The hair is then dried. The dye coats the hair only and is easily washed out with the next shampoo. You will find a caution notice of some type present on the package.

Advantages: This is a product of very low cost.

Disadvantages: Only a limited color range with minimal depth is possible. You can only darken your hair with this product. It produces some blending of grey, but does not cover it well.

Although easily washed out, significant residual staining of grey, white or very blonde hair may occur to make future use of other dye products complicated. Fading takes place in the sun and with excessive perspiration to distort the tone and produce an unnatural color.

7. METALLIC DYES are made available in liquid, lotion or pomade form. A small quantity of the preparation is repeatedly applied directly to the hair with the fingers or with a comb. No immediate color change takes place. With the passage of time, the air slowly acts upon the dye material which in turn reacts with the outer coating of the hair to produce a gradual darkening. Label instructions usually recommend that daily application be discontinued when the desired degree of darkening has been achieved. No skin patch test is required.

Advantages: These dyes produce slow, gradual results. It has good acceptance by men who are particularly eager to avoid startling change.

Disadvantages: It is only possible to darken hair, in a very limited shade range, with such products. Color builds up with use, often to an unnatural brassy and occasionally coppery-green metallic tone. Color distortion also occurs following exposure to sun and excessive perspiration. It is difficult to remove the color should the future use of other dye products be attempted. The alteration that occurs in hair shaft structure demands great caution if permanent waving or straightening preparations are to be used. For the same reason, care must be exercised with other manipulative procedures such as hair teasing.

8. THE VEGETABLE RINSES such as henna or camomile deserve no discussion. Their quality of performance is so poor and their use so rare that they are all but impossible to obtain in most communities.

Hair Waving

As previously mentioned, the hair shaft is almost entirely protein. Proteins are very complicated and large chemical molecules. Smaller chemical molecules, let us call them building blocks, are intricately bunched or joined together in the formation of the protein molecule. Many protein molecules are then linked together, in special fashion, to form the visible substance we call protein. The particular building blocks that are selected, the number that are chosen, and the pattern with which they are joined together account for the differences between proteins. Egg white is pure protein as is also gelatin.

Heat and certain chemicals, by acting upon the points of linkage between the protein molecules, cause the protein substance to take on an altered physical appearance, usually of a permanent nature. This is called denaturization. The solidified hard-boiled egg is a typical example of permanently altered physical characteristics of a certain protein following the application of heat; tanned leather is an example of permanently altered physical characteristics of a certain protein (animal skin) by chemical means.

In similar fashion, the physical appearance of the special protein substance which makes up the hair can be changed. Curl or roll the hair in a desired position; apply heat which alters (softens, in this case), the hair's chemical structure; allow to cool in the new position. The hair will take on its new shape just as the egg white will conform to the position into which it is molded as it is poured into a hot frying pan.

This is the very principle upon which the warmed rollers, the curling iron, the hot comb, etc. all work. The more heat that is applied to the hair the greater is the structural alteration in its protein molecules and the more permanent will its new shape be—curled or straightened. Too much heat can cause so great a structural chemical alteration that the hair shaft will produce an undesirable "frizzy" appearance. It may break off. This can also happen if lesser degrees of heat are applied too frequently to the same portions of the hair. However, *no matter what the alteration to the hair shaft, there is no influence upon the growing capacity of the hair.* The hair bulb continues to function. As new hair grows out, it is normal in every way and will withstand further alteration by heat, as previously.

In the early days of the "hot wave permanent," it was found that pretreating the hair with certain chemicals prior to the application of heat considerably improved the quality and permanency of the wave. Before the adaptation of electric heating pads, it was clumsy and extremely time-consuming to heat individual curled sections of hair for adequate periods.

Even with newer electric devices, just getting set into the equipment required considerable time and skilled attention. The method was just too restrictive to have wide appeal. These elaborate waving machines are now just memories.

The all-chemical "cold waving" process for permanent waving began in the 1930's and the method was remarkably improved after World War II. The procedure is simple, quick, requires no special apparatus, and produces excellent results. These products have also been modified for home use; their speed of action and overall effectiveness has been reduced for easy handling by the casual user.

Basic Principles for Best Results

Even though you may never wave your own hair, you may be interested in the principle. It will help you understand the procedure. You will know what can and what cannot be accomplished. You will also know what can go wrong and why.

If you enjoy doing things to your hair—or a friend's—then the basic facts that follow are must reading. You cannot approach the task of waving, straightening or coloring your hair with the same attitude you have in following a new cake recipe. You just can't throw out your mistakes and bad judgment and begin all over again whenever you choose.

All consumer products, and particularly hair coloring, waving and straightening items, are carefully tested and retested by the manufacturer. Each step in the directions is checked and rechecked. In my experience, unhappy results are always caused by failure to follow directions: steps are omitted, shortcuts are taken, variations are made in the procedure. *Do not do it!*

Each product has its own specific directions; the following is merely a general description of the method.

After being freshly washed, section your hair into blocks approximately ½ to 1 inch by 2 to 3 inches in dimension. Comb out these blocks of hair and apply waving lotion lightly. Then wind the hair around a curler. "End papers" are usually used to collect together the hair ends to facilitate winding onto the curler. The wound hair is then fixed in position with a clip, bobby pin or similar device. Additional waving lotion is then applied to the wound hair.

The success of the waving procedure depends upon the following important factors:

1. The degree of physical alteration exerted upon the hair shaft. This means the number of turns or windings the hair shaft makes upon the curler. With a bigger curler diameter, fewer complete windings will be possible than with a narrow curler. The narrow curler will, therefore, make a tighter wave.

2. It takes one full wrapping of hair about the curler to make a *half wave* in your hair shaft. Therefore, you must have sufficient hair length for winding about the curler before you can expect success.

3. As the bulk amount of hair increases on the curler, less physical alteration is exerted upon the section of hair shaft that is rolled up last. Since you wind from the ends toward the scalp, it is the hair closest to the scalp that is waved least. To quickly understand this physical principle, roll up a sheet of stiff typewriter paper. The inside of the roll is tightest. When you unravel the paper, that section of the paper will have the "tighter," more pronounced curl. Therefore, hair length is an important consid-

eration. It may be too short for a good wind, or so long that only the outer sections will get a good wave.

4. The portion of the hair strand that is closest to the curler (the inside portion) gets more strain than the outer portion as it is wound on the curler. With coarse hair, this effect is much greater than with fine hair. It is similar to rolling up sheets of paper. Thin, soft paper will unroll to almost its original flatness. Coarse, stiff paper will keep a wave in it even after you try to unravel it. Therefore, the coarser your hair, the more definite a curl you can expect.

5. The more perfect the outermost coating of your hair shaft (the cuticle), the greater will its resistance be to the effects of the waving chemical. Previously waved, bleached or tinted hair has tiny breaks in its outer coating. Such hair is more porous. It will easily accept and be affected by the waving solution. This is why a child's hair, with its perfect cuticle, is always so much more difficult to wave than an adult's.

6. The strength (concentration) of the waving solution and the time it is allowed to act upon the hair determine the amount of physical change that can be produced upon your hair. But you must also take into account all the other factors enumerated above.

The waving solution, an acid (thioglycolic), which saturates your wound hair, actually "softens" the protein of the hair filament. Your hair molecules can now rearrange themselves to conform to the new position—the windings about the curler. Considering all the principles enumerated above, the proper concentration of waving solution is left in place for the time required to achieve satisfactory results.

The waving lotion is either blotted up or rinsed out with water and a chemical neutralizer is applied to the curled hair. This step fixes the hair filaments in their new shape and stops further action of the waving solution. After several minutes, the hair is thoroughly rinsed with water, taken down and set and dried in the usual manner.

One-step, self-neutralizing waving lotions are also available; because of their simplicity of use, they are particularly advantageous for the unskilled individual to use at home. These preparations contain a special chemical (a catalyst) that allows the air itself to neutralize the waving lotion. The hair, therefore, is "softened" and "fixed" in one procedure. Some manufacturers recommend blotting the lotion from the wound hair after a specified time period has elapsed. This allows air better access to the rolled hair for greater efficiency. Instructions vary from one product to another. When the full time period specified by the manufacturer has elapsed, the hair is then rinsed with water, taken down and set and dried in the usual manner.

The two-step waving method as well as the self-neutralizing preparations are usually available to the consumer in three strengths, depending upon your hair texture. They are weaker in concentration than the waving lotions used by the professional. The action of air as a neutralizer is also a slower process than chemical neutralization. Consequently, the self-neutralizing products are not suitable for salon use.

Hair waving, whether performed at home or in a salon, can achieve highly desirable and attractive results. The professional operator will often perform a test curl to determine what procedure will give the best results. For home use, package directions must be carefully read and followed. The test curl is a very important guide. If any hair breakage occurs on the test curl, it is best that the amateur not continue with the procedure at all.

It is a good idea to schedule this kind of self-care when you can devote the time and attention to details. Scampering children or a busy telephone do not allow for careful concentration. Remember that hair texture and quality vary from person to person. The product and method that produce satisfactory results for you may not do the same for your neighbor.

When undesirable results take place, there is a reasonable explanation for them:

Reasons for Failures

1. A poor wave or "take": This may be caused by a solution that is too weak, or one not left in contact with the hair long enough to soften the hair before neutralization. With young or virginal hair having a very intact cuticle, this dissatisfaction is especially common. Soiled hair or hair with a very high degree of oil incompletely washed out will also resist the waving action and result in a poor take.

2. Scant wave with no body: Hair that is too short for at least one full turn on the curler, or hair that is not wound tightly enough about the curler to create adequate stress upon the hair filament, will cause a scant or limp wave.

3. Only ends of hair curled well: Hair that is very long may be too bulky on the roller. Adequate stress is created only on the portion of the shafts that are closest to the surface of the curlers.

4. Frizzy or wire-like texture (steel-wool effect): This is caused by too much hair curled

too strongly. You may have made too many curls. Or, if your hair is long, too much hair was taken up on rollers that were too narrow (diameter not big enough). Each long hair shaft acquired more than one complete wave (more than two complete turns of the roller). Overcurled or tightly curled hair produces a frizzy effect.

5. Excessive hair breakage: Caused by too much chemical action on the hair. The waving solution may have been too strong. Perhaps for the texture and quality of your hair, the timing was excessively long. Waving methods that worked well for you previously must be revised if used at frequent intervals or in association with other hair altering techniques such as bleaching and tinting.

6. Scalp sores or skin irritation: The waving solution can be irritating to skin. It should not contact the skin. Be careful to confine the solution to the wound hair only. If the skin of your scalp is not in a healthy state, it is a wise precaution to avoid using hair-waving chemicals until it has recovered.

Hair waving, as with bleaching and toning, produces a measure of irreversible chemical and structural change to your hair filaments. Such hair requires careful attention in future washing, combing and styling. Its ability to withstand ordinary manipulation, easily tolerated previously, has been reduced. As new hair grows out, however, it is as strong and healthy as ever. For the most satisfactory results, you should limit permanent hair waving to two or three times per year.

If you desire to both color and wave your hair, separate the procedure by as long a time (in days) as convenience permits. Schedule with foresight. It is absence of planning, lack of understanding, or willful disregard of established protocol that is responsible for the regrettable, but avoidable, mishaps that occasionally take place.

The mother of the bride will plan her daughter's wedding reception in minute detail and follow through to the writing of the last place card. She remembers to make an appointment at the beauty salon for the very week-end of the wedding, if possible. She insists. After all, it is such a special event.

At 10 A.M. Mrs. Busymother arrives at a salon already crowded with other women who also must look their best for the week-end. She informs the operator she wants to be exotic— new hair style—new color. Some time later the operator is advised that Mrs. Busymother is also planning to meet her sister's plane from St. Louis at 2 P.M.! There's no time for a patch test! She protests "Wasn't it O.K. once? I didn't let you do it last time, and there was no problem. Besides I'm as strong as a horse." This lady is not interested in a mere touch-up. She wants to "go lighter." A thorough bleaching of hair color is necessary before application of the toner.

Mrs. Busymother grows alarmed at all the time it is taking. Every operator in the salon becomes involved; frenetic phone calls interrupt the hair coloring to arrange for someone else to meet the plane from St. Louis. Confusion reigns supreme. Yet, Mrs. Busymother remains deaf to reason. Her hair must also be waved! At least a little bit! It's now she wants to look her best, not next week. The wedding is tomorrow!

It is pressure, pressure, pressure, cutting corners, compromise, and contempt for proper and established practice. It sets the stage for skin irritation or regrettable hair damage, disappointment and despair. Under the proper circumstances, safety and satisfaction can be and are consistently and easily achieved. Mrs. Busymother is not fair to herself, her beauty salon, or the wonderful products and procedures designed for her pleasure.

Straightening Hair

The mechanisms for straightening or, more accurately, relaxing natural hair curl are the same as those for inducing a wave. The protein structure of the hair filament is altered in either a temporary or permanent fashion so that it will conform to an artificially produced configuration. In this instance, however, the new configuration is to uncurl it, to try to make it as straight as possible.

There are, of course, temporary methods for straightening hair that do not change the physico-chemical properties of the hair. They are waxes and gums, dressings that stiffen the hair filament with an outside coating. They are of value only on short hair. Their greatest popularity has been as mustache wax, training compounds for the wayward strands of boys' hair, and to create certain square-shaped crewcut hair styles. Water quickly removes this dressed effect.

The oldest, simplest, and most common method for straightening the hair is heat. As explained previously, heat is an excellent means for denaturing protein. Instead of an "iron," shaped to curl, a heated metal comb is pulled through the hair, heating and stretching out the strands to achieve a straightened shape. Freshly washed and thoroughly dried hair responds best. The application of oil or petrolatum makes it easier to pull the heated comb through the hair strands, and especially aids in conducting heat to the hair filaments to improve efficiency. You must acquire skill to produce satisfactory straightening of the hair without singeing it. Electrically heated combs reduce this risk. Unfortunately, the altered shape of the hair strand produced by the hot comb is not permanent. Time and moisture soon return the strand to its natural position.

I have recently learned that many teenage girls, in their quest for ever straighter hair, have devised their own method. A friend combs and spreads another's hair over a laundry ironing board; it is then covered with a sheet of waxed paper and pressed with a warm laundry iron. The heat and pressure of the iron straightens out the hair filaments. They also become coated with a thin layer of wax from the paper to help "set" or stiffen each filament. Successful temporary straightening can be achieved in some instances. However, the crudeness of the method exposes these youngsters to dangerous hazard.

As you would expect, the same family of chemicals (thioglycolates) found best for producing a permanent wave, serve equally well for permanent straightening. This is the chemical method for denaturing the hair protein. Since such products can only lessen the natural wave rather than yield straight hair, they are labeled "curl relaxers." The principle is the same as in waving hair. The method is somewhat more involved. Products are available for home use if you choose not to seek professional attention.

As discussed in an earlier section on waving, inherited qualities of hair, plus any acquired alteration in outer structure, such as the tiny breaks in the cuticle surface associated with tinting and bleaching, will influence the response of the hair to the straightening solution. To determine how your hair will respond, the entire straightening procedure (including final drying of the hair) should be performed on a strand of hair first. The non-professional must always do this strand test. If you are not satisfied with the feel of the strand or its appearance, then your hair should not be straightened by this method. For example, it may feel rubbery or gummy when wet; wiry and brittle as it dries. It may show excessive breakage or become discolored. Heed such signs carefully and do not continue with the procedure.

Since the chemicals themselves may be irritating to skin, these preparations should be avoided if the skin of the scalp is abraded or otherwise unhealthy. In like fashion, the hands should be protected with rubber or plastic gloves.

The following description of the method is given not as directions, but to illustrate the intricacies and explain some of the details. Thoroughly shampoo the hair to remove soil, oil or any coating that might interfere with the chemical reaction. Blot dry and comb free of tangles. The straightening lotion (previously mixed and allowed to stand for ten to fifteen minutes) is now liberally applied to the hair, avoiding contact with the skin. Spread the lotion over the hair with the fingers. In a systematic fashion, beginning at the neck and working upward, the hair of the entire scalp is covered generously with lotion. Great care must be taken to moisten all surfaces of the hair, under as well as upper. Then comb the hair gently and wrap in a plastic turban for ten to twenty minutes to permit the solution to soften the hair filaments.

Following removal of the turban, gently comb the hair through its complete length and over the entire scalp. This step of the procedure is very important. It is with the combing of the chemically denatured hair filaments that the natural curl of the hair is being straightened or re-positioned. Consequently, this combing must be deliberate and continuous for ten to twenty minutes.

Rinse the hair thoroughly with liberal amounts of lukewarm water. A spray device is advisable. Blot well and once more comb free of tangles. A neutralizing lotion (previously mixed and allowed to stand) is now just as thoroughly and carefully applied to the hair as the original hair straightening lotion. Every attempt should be made to keep the hair shafts straight and free of tangles. The neutralizer should remain on the hair for five minutes and then thoroughly rinsed with lukewarm water.

After blotting with a towel, your hair may be set and styled to preference. The approximate time for the above (exclusive of setting and styling) is two hours. This straightening procedure, like permanent waving, should be repeated only when new hair growth has taken place to require it.

If you are dissatisfied with the results, there is always a reasonable explanation.

VERY LITTLE AND INADEQUATE STRAIGHTENING: This may be caused by solutions that are too weak, hair that is incompletely saturated; or inadequate time before application of the neutralizer. The straightener solution must be applied to all surfaces of the shaft and then combed through completely. Young or virginal hair with a very intact cuticle, or soiled hair with a very high degree of oil (incompletely washed out prior to the application of straightener solution) may resist the chemical action.

WIRY OR BRITTLE HAIR when it is dry or a gummy, rubbery texture when it is wet: The straightening solution produced too much change in the chemistry of the hair shaft. Solutions that are too strong, or left in place too long for your hair quality, are usually the cause. It is also possible that your hair was bleached and toned recently. The time interval between procedures was too short. When this occurs the hair shafts acquire numerous breaks in the cuticle surface. When dry it is very brittle. Such hair is very porous; it takes up water almost like a sponge to give the hair a gummy or rubbery feel when wet.

EXCESSIVE HAIR BREAKAGE is also the result of too much chemical action on the hair, either from the straightening procedure itself or when performed too soon after other hair altering techniques, as bleaching and toning. Remember, the physical condition of your hair at the time you plan to straighten your hair is an important consideration. The procedure that worked well for you in times past may not suit the present situation. This is why the strand test is such a valuable guide and an absolute requirement if you are an amateur.

SCALP SORES OR SKIN IRRITATION may result from lotion contacting the skin and remaining on it for too long a time. Work as neatly as possible. Avoid soiling the skin and blot up solution that comes in contact with it. It is a wise precaution to avoid hair straightening products if the skin of the scalp is not in a healthy state.

Hair straightening, like waving, bleaching and toning, produces a measure of irreversible chemical and structural change to your hair filaments. Such hair requires careful attention in future washing, combing and styling. Its ability to withstand ordinary manipulation, easily tolerated previously, has been reduced. As new hair grows out, however, it is as strong and healthy as ever.

Excessive Hair (Hirsutism)

As mentioned in an early chapter on hair growth, some type of hair is present everywhere on the skin, except for the palms, soles and mucous membranes. Over some surfaces it may be fine, flesh-colored, downy in texture and almost invisible.

The greatest change in hair distribution and appearance occurs at puberty. While the teenage boy admires the advancing and darkening hairs that appear in clusters about the sides of his face, upper lip, chin, armpits and chest, the teenage girl views with horror the slightest prominence of any hair on such critical surfaces of her own body.

In both instances the phenomenon is normal. It is caused by the increase in body hormones produced at adolescence. In our society, however, the hair growth on the girl is considered undesirable, unflattering, unwanted, and—to her—excessive. As birthdays go by, the hairs may increase in number, even grow darker and more prominent. Other body surfaces as the arms, legs and even the chest present increased amounts of hair. Although normal, it is unacceptable to many of us because of the demands of our society.

A few rare internal diseases may cause an

increase in body hair. However, while the physician is investigating and treating such internal disorders, the cosmetic problem created by the excessive hair growth can be improved by the very measures described in this section.

For our purposes, then, the definition of excessive hair simply means any hair growth (normal or abnormal) appearing anywhere on the body, which the individual herself (or himself) deems undesirable. This includes a desire to change the configuration of eyebrows, the hairline about the upper forehead, the more mature woman's objection to the coarse dark hairs sprinkled about her face, as well as the universal female objection to the hair on the extremities.

Many methods are available for correcting the undesirable appearance of excessive hair. The method you select will depend much upon the effort and cost you are ready to assume, the skin area involved, and the amount and color of the hair to be eliminated. Consequently, you will probably find it expedient to select several methods for the control of your excessive hair. All the methods will be fully discussed along with the skin surfaces for which they are best suited.

Methods for the Removal of Hair (Depilatories)

SHAVING. This is the first considered and most commonly used method for removing excessive hair; millions of men the world over practice it as a daily ritual. The procedure is simple; the materials required are few and readily available; adequate skill is quickly acquired to yield fast results with little hazard. The surface to be shaved is washed with soap and water to remove oils as well as soil. Cleansing the skin reduces the chance of infection if the skin is nicked. Freeing the hair of oil permits water to penetrate, soften, and swell each shaft to make it stand free for easier shaving. Warm water performs better than cold. The application of lather is the easiest and most efficient way to keep the hair and skin moist. A multitude of modern shaving foams, creams, and soaps are available to make this a simple and convenient task.

Equip your safety razor (straight razors are for the experts), with a sharp blade; place it against the skin and draw it across the hairy surface in long, deliberate, but gentle strokes, preferably in the opposite direction to which the hair grows. Flush the razor frequently with clear water to avoid clogging the cutting channel. When you have shaved off all the hair, cleanse and dry the skin surface. If you nicked the skin, a few moments of continuous firm pressure with a clean dry cloth or facial tissue will usually stop bleeding. For rapid results, touch the bleeding spot with the moistened tip of a styptic pencil. This is a stick of a highly astringent chemical which promotes the clotting of blood from tiny wounds.

Many women use a dry shave technique—no lather. It is an inferior method. I believe it is preferred by women who consider it too masculine to apply a lather. The dry procedure, being different, seems to have less stigma. There is no doubt that visibility is better when lather is absent. Whatever advantage this offers is more than offset by its many deficiencies.

Electric razors in cord as well as cordless varieties have been designed for shaving the face as well as other skin surfaces. They yield very good results. Your skin surface should be free of moisture. Pre-electric shave lotions prepare the hair and skin surface for efficient performance of these devices.

Advantages: Any large skin surface can be quickly denuded of hair. No special skill is required, and it can be self-performed with ease. Shaving may be repeated as often as necessary and at minimal cost.

Misconceptions: Although persistent chronic irritation over a circumscribed surface area has been known to increase hair growth (this is probably hair length rather than number of hairs in a given area), there is no valid medical evidence that regular shaving causes more hair to grow. What is a fact is that the original condition which causes your excessive hair remains present to permit and cause more new hair to grow with the passage of time. This phenomenon would have taken place even if no method for hair removal was practiced. It has been convenient but erroneous to relate the progression of new hair growth to shaving.

Disadvantages: As your hair regrows, the short shafts (stubble) that appear above the skin surface are stiff. This conveys a coarse, spiny and undesirable feel to the skin. As hair length increases, the filaments regain their usual flexibility and softness. It is not true that shaving makes the hair coarse and dark.

In shaved bearded areas of dense hair growth only, men may notice a bluish color to the skin surface. This is caused by the very dark hair within each follicle. The hair pigment, deep in the skin, imparts a steel-blue color. Although shaving off the surface hair allows you to see this color, shaving does not make the color.

Even with great care, nicks and small cuts may occur which, if not properly cared for, particularly in susceptible individuals, may lead to infection or persistent local skin inflammation. This is of particular concern over the legs as normal blood circulation becomes deficient with age and the healing process is retarded.

WAXING. A depilatory wax is a mixture of several types of waxes, oils and resins. It has a solid consistency at body temperature; however, when it is warmed to a temperature that is still tolerable to the skin, the wax is a liquid or semi-solid. The heated, softened wax is spread over the hairy surface in a thin strip; as it cools, it hardens. The hair shafts become firmly embedded in this hardened wax. One end of the strip is grasped tightly and with one quick, deliberate motion, peeled off the skin. Ripped off is probably more descriptive. This sharp motion of the wax with the hairs embedded within it actually pulls each hair out of its follicle to produce a smooth and hair-free surface. The principle is exactly the same as quickly tearing off a strip of adhesive tape from a hairy surface. Adhesive tape is not as efficient because the molten wax enmeshes the hair shafts better than the tape to leave little or no hair behind as it is stripped off.

Advantages: The method is quick and efficient, particularly for large, flat, hairy areas. Since the hair is pulled out from deep in the follicle, as compared to being shaved off at the skin surface, the period of time elapsing between treatments is longer.

Disadvantages: It is difficult to do this procedure properly to yourself. Some pain is experienced even at the hands of the most skilled operator. Occasionally some of the follicles will ooze a drop of blood. It works well only over flat skin surfaces such as the legs or portions of the face. It cannot be used in the armpits or for fine work, such as shaping eyebrows or hairline.

TWEEZING. This is merely pulling out hairs individually from the follicle. Success depends on the use of an instrument that is made with precision; the tweezer ends must meet perfectly to permit a firm hold upon the isolated hair. Be sure the steel shafts of the instrument you select are not too flexible and terminate in a flat working surface rather than sharp points. Poorly designed, cheap tweezers are exasperating to use. Your well-lighted, magnifying make-up mirror and the make-up glasses described in Chapter VIII will simplify your task immeasurably.

Wash the area to be tweezed with soap and water; then cleanse with alcohol. Grasp a single hair only with the tweezers; pull firmly and quickly, out and away, from the skin surface *but at the same angle from which the hair grows out of the skin surface.* You will then be certain of removing the hair in depth from the follicle rather than merely breaking it off at the skin surface. Properly removed hair will take longer to regrow. Be sure to keep the tweezer surfaces free of hair and debris to assure a good grip upon the next hair. Dip the instrument in alcohol from time to time. When you have completed tweezing an area, cleanse the skin surface with alcohol. Such care will reduce the chance for an infection.

Advantages: This is a simple, easily performed method requiring little skill; you can do it yourself. Discomfort is minimal. It is excellent for removing the isolated troublesome hairs about the face as well as for performing fine detailed shaping of eyebrows.

Disadvantages: It is far too slow and uncomfortable a procedure for large hairy surfaces. Wax depilation is really the "tweezing" of such areas.

ABRASIVE DEPILATORIES.   Roughened waxes or sandpaper-like cloth, fashioned into a mitt, are available for lightly rubbing the skin surface. By doing so you actually wear down or cut off the hair without injuring the skin. There is no discomfort.

It appears to have no advantage over ordinary shaving. It is practical only for surfaces that are large and flat with considerable quantities of hair.

BLEACHING.   You may find that you can achieve a very satisfactory improvement in appearance by merely bleaching your excessive hair. You are simply reducing the color contrast between your skin and the hair. The excessive hair about your upper lip and legs are particularly suited for bleaching.

Ordinary peroxide that is used for cleansing minor cuts and wounds is not strong enough to bleach hair. You must use beauticians' (twenty volume, six percent) peroxide freshly prepared with ammonia, about twenty drops per ounce of peroxide. Saturate a cloth and apply for twenty to thirty minutes.

The bleach products especially designed for bleaching scalp hair will work very satisfactorily elsewhere provided you practice care in the application of the material and in its timing. These products contain hydrogen peroxide and an activator powder or liquid which mix into a thick lotion that will not run or drip off your skin. Apply the freshly prepared mixture to the surface to be bleached. Allow to remain in place just long enough to decolorize the hair. Rinse off thoroughly with fresh water. The treatment time will vary with your hair color and its texture. First test an area one inch in diameter to determine both your skin tolerance to the bleach substance and the time required (usually twenty to thirty minutes) for achieving the best results. If you experience skin discomfort or irritation, do not continue with this procedure.

Advantages: Once hair has grown to its full length for a particular skin surface, it enters into a resting stage which may last for weeks or months. When this hair is shed, breaks, or wears off, a newly grown hair takes its place. Consequently, fully grown bleached hair over the legs or upper lip does not require rebleaching more than a few times a year. The method produces quick results and avoids the unpleasant regrowth stubble that follows shaving.

Disadvantages: Bleaching does not remove hair; it only makes it less conspicuous. Consequently, it will not please the woman who insists on a hairless skin surface for such areas as the armpits and the face. These bleaching chemicals must not be used about your eyes; avoid them completely if your skin cannot tolerate them.

CHEMICAL DEPILATORIES. These are creams, lotions, pastes or foams that contain chemicals which soften hair protein. The chemical reaction is permitted to continue until the hair can actually be wiped off the skin with a cloth. The principle of protein denaturization is now carried to an extreme in order to destroy the excess hair.

Formerly, these products depended upon a family of chemicals called metallic sulfides. They were easily recognized by the strong and very unpleasant odor of rotten eggs that accompanied their use. The modern chemical depilatories produce little odor. Their basic ingredient is a thioglycolate—similar to the same chemical used to wave hair. However, in depilatory form it is used in greater strength, without a neutralization step, in order to achieve protein softening that permits the hair to be wiped off.

Since the protein of hair and skin is similar, chemical depilatories must be used with care and understanding to avoid irritation to the skin; consequently, you must follow the manufacturer's directions in every detail.

Skin surfaces that have cuts or abrasions, or that are otherwise not healthy, should not receive chemical depilatories. Remember that your normal-looking skin can be irritated by or may be sensitive to the chemicals in the product. You can easily determine this by performing a simple preliminary test.

To an easily accessible area of skin, about one inch in diameter, apply the depilatory and let it remain in place as directed by the manufacturer (usually five to ten minutes); then wash off thoroughly. Wait twenty-four hours and examine the test area carefully. If redness or irritation is present, you must not use the product. If the test area is free of any reaction, you may proceed to use the depilatory over the skin surfaces from which you desire to remove the hair. Allow it to remain in place only as long as the manufacturer directs (usually five to ten minutes); wipe off the skin surface with a damp cloth and cleanse with fresh water.

Advantages: It is easy and quick; it can be self-performed. If used as directed, it is safe. Large or small body surfaces can be treated regardless of their contour. The process can be repeated each time the hair returns. Since the hair is removed slightly deeper in the hair follicle than with shaving, hair regrowth takes a little longer following chemical depilation than shaving. As with shaving, the repeated use of chemical depilatories does not increase the problem of excessive hair.

Disadvantages: Chemical depilatories are not designed for use about the eyes. Accidental insertion can cause damage to the eye. Individuals with skin sensitivity to such chemicals must avoid them. Hair regrowth after chemical depilation has the same unpleasant rough, spiny stubble that is so undesirable following shaving. If you permit the hair shafts to grow longer, they regain flexibility and their usual texture.

Except for bleaching, all of the above procedures provide a *temporary removal* of hair from the skin surface. Shaving, waxing and chemical depilation are not selective. They remove all the hair—the fine, almost imperceptible downy hair, as well as the coarse, dark, and obviously excessive hair. It is this total loss of the downy hair fuzz that makes the skin look shiny and marble-like. Light striking the smooth skin surface is reflected as from a slab of polished stone. With hair regrowth, a more normal light-reflectance pattern returns.

ELECTROLYSIS. Let us now discuss a method of hair removal that is not only permanent but highly selective—only the excessive or undesirable hair is removed. The fine down is left to convey a natural, desirable, and attractive skin appearance. The method is generally known as electrolysis. It is worthy of special discussion and consideration.

The medical or surgical meaning of electrolysis is the alteration of tissue by means of an electric current. The type of current (direct, low voltage and low amperage) and its method of application produce unique effects. Some fundamental chemical constituents of living tissue become rearranged and actually migrate in the body between the electrodes or poles of the electrical circuit.

If a needle is one of the electrodes, the rearrangement of body chemicals will result in the deposition of tiny amounts of a caustic or an acid at the needle point, depending upon whether the electrode is negatively or positively charged. As you know from previous discussions, these chemicals, even though minute in amount, will cause protein to become denatured. If the needle is left in place for a long enough period of time, sufficient caustic or acid is produced to destroy minuscule amounts of living tissue protein. This simple machine, with its negatively charged needle electrode, becomes ideally suited for fine, detailed work—such as the destruction of individual hairs.

The needle of the electrolysis machine is finer than a hair filament. The operator, following the direction in which the hair grows, inserts this needle into the hair follicle opening on the skin. The skilled operator can easily feel when the needle point reaches the base of the hair— the actual root or growing portion of the hair. The electric current is then applied to produce the necessary caustic material at the needle point for destruction of the hair root.

The insertion of the needle into the hair follicle is completely painless; however, as the caustic chemical is formed, a stinging, but tolerable, sensation is felt at the site of treatment.

The destructive chemical forms slowly. It may take as long as a minute for sufficient caustic to be deposited to destroy a single hair root. The current is then turned off and the hair is removed by the operator with a pair of tweezers. The properly destroyed hair offers no resistance to the tug of the tweezers. The hair is withdrawn as easily as if it were being pulled out of petroleum jelly.

Because of the great time required to destroy each hair, some operators work with machines that have many needles. Each is inserted in sequence. By the time the last needle has been placed, it is time to withdraw the first, remove the hair, replace it in another follicle, and continue on.

The electrolysis machine, for practical reasons, has been replaced by the *high-frequency* machine. A similar needle is inserted into the hair follicle in exactly the same manner as previously; however, it is connected to an electrical device which produces energy of the diathermy type (actually long radio waves) at the needle tip. When the current is turned on, a momentary minute blast of this energy about the needle point heats up the tissue to destroy it. It takes but a second, or less. The hair itself is easily removed with the tweezers. A minor degree of discomfort, quite tolerable, is experienced at the brief moment when the current is applied.

This modern equipment is, technically speaking, not electrolysis. However, this name, by custom, is generally used to describe the electrical method for the permanent removal of hair.

The skilled operator works very rapidly with this high-frequency equipment and can destroy hundreds of hairs in a fifteen-minute period. You will easily tolerate any minor discomfort. Like most individuals, you will readily accept fifteen to thirty or more minutes of treatment without difficulty.

The treatment is not confined to an isolated area of skin—even if the program is to remove only the hair over your upper lip. The operator will, instead, skip around over the entire lip area during each treatment period. There are two very good reasons for doing this: (1) To completely remove all the hair from a confined zone would produce an obvious and unattractive effect—excessive hair on the left but not the right, or clearing under the nose at the expense of both sides of the lip! By skillfully skipping about, a gradual, non-eye-catching effect takes place; (2) the tissue actually destroyed by the treatment to each hair is so infinitesimal that your body's healing process recovers without any perceptible scarring. However, to treat many hairs in one confined area during a single treatment period without sufficient time for recovery is to risk connecting many tiny areas of fresh destruction into a large one—one that could be capable of healing with visible scarring.

Within twenty-four hours of a treatment, you may experience red and even tender tiny elevations about the treated hair openings. This is a common healing response for many. Complete, uneventful recovery will follow within a few days.

Electrolysis is a method for the *permanent* removal of hair. Good scientific investigation has repeatedly shown that eighty out of every hundred hairs so treated are permanently destroyed, never to return. Twenty do return. They are not destroyed because the operator, no matter how experienced, cannot administer just enough current at the proper location in the hair follicle every time. No matter how experienced the seamstress, needle-threading may occasionally require a second try! Another, and probably more contributory, cause to account for some hairs avoiding destruction is their presence in a resting phase of growth at the time of treatment. A certain small percentage of the hair population at any time is in a resting stage. When in this stage, the hairs are particularly resistant to electrolysis. Fortunately, the next time these hairs come under treatment, the odds are all against their surviving and their permanent removal is achieved.

With a regular, frequent and faithfully maintained program of electrolysis, remarkable results can be achieved even if you have severe excessive hair growth. I can recall several instances of weeping, mature as well as young, women who appeared in my office. Their faces were almost completely hidden by kerchiefs. They wept out of grief and veiled their faces to society. They were hiding hair growth on the face as heavy as found on some men. Periodic shaving was necessary to afford them some freedom of movement in their limited world. With hardly more than a year of treatment, these women were returning to a normal existence—the joy of free social contacts and gainful employment. Disfiguring hair was permanently removed as a result of electrolysis. More grateful patients cannot be found in any practice.

Whether you have a minor or a major excessive hair problem that has been successfully treated by electrolysis, remember that the underlying cause has not, in any way, been affected by electrolysis. The destroyed follicles can never produce another hair; however, previously dormant and untreated follicles may begin to grow hair. This would have happened even if you received no electrolysis. This is not a failure of the method; don't lose confidence in it. Treatment of this new growth, at occasional and infrequent intervals, will quickly maintain the status you desire.

Hair on any body surface may be removed by electrolysis. It is not possible to predict the degree of discomfort you will experience. Generally speaking, the upper lip is most sensitive to the stinging sensation, and the legs the least. As you gain confidence in the operator and the method, none of the stinging seems to matter at all.

Because of the fine details of the procedure, it is possible to perform remarkable effects in shaping eyebrows and hairline. Isolated or clusters of coarse hairs are easily removed from the chest, about the nipples, or from any region you wish denuded.

The operator (or electrologist) must be able to see each hair and its direction of growth and be able to grasp it with a tweezer before destruction is possible. Consequently, you must allow your excessive hair to grow sufficiently, about ⅛ to ¼ inch, before submitting yourself to electrolysis. This will permit an evaluation of your total problem. It will be possible to determine your reaction to the procedure itself following the removal of a few test hairs from various sites. Then, you can decide on the frequency of treatments, based on your tolerance of the discomfort as well as their cost. Only with this information can a minimum estimate be made of the total time that will be necessary to achieve satisfaction.

These can only be very rough estimates. Individuals differ widely in their reaction to the procedure, the amount of time they will give to each treatment, and the degree of cooperation offered to the operator. Since this is not a method that can be self-performed, its cost is often a serious limiting factor.

Obviously, it is very important that you select a good electrologist. The technique is easily learned by any reasonably adept individual. Several teaching centers across the country have excellent short courses for training electrologists. A physician can train a technician in his office in a matter of hours.

Unfortunately, many states of the United States do not require the licensing of electrologists. While most operators are excellent and reliable, it is best to have some prior knowledge of their reputation before accepting their services. Your own physician, particularly your dermatologist, will be able to help you most. He may have a technician that performs this service in his own office or know one or more electrologists in your community upon whose ability and reliability he has learned to depend.

From time to time magazine and newspaper advertisements appear featuring a pen-sized electrolysis machine for personal home use. It is indeed capable of destroying hair roots if properly used. Because of its design it will only work upon the individual who is holding it. It will not work if one person is attempting to treat another unless special adapters are acquired. The successful performance of electrolysis depends upon many important maneuvers: good visibility of the area to be treated; the ability to focus down to a single hair follicle; the dexterity to insert a fine needle; holding it steady for almost a minute (since this is a true old-style electrolysis unit); concentrating on treated hair so that it can be grasped by the tweezers for removal.

An expert electrologist to whom I gave such a gadget found it possible to treat the hair on accessible areas of her left arm (since she's right-handed) and legs. Due to the time required for destroying a single hair, it was hardly practical for treating more than an isolated hair. It was difficult and all but impossible for this expert to treat the hairs of her face where the problem is exaggerated by the optical confusion of mirror movements.

Electrolysis is an excellent method for the permanent removal of hair. It is a procedure to be carried out only by properly trained individuals.

The Ingrown Hair

Very rarely, when a hair has been plucked or tweezed or shaved off, the uppermost portions of the outer skin layer (epidermis) may grow over and cover the normal hair opening. As the hair regrows, it is unable to push its way through the skin which has roofed over its channel. The hair, therefore, coils on itself as it continues to grow. It balls up. This ingrown hair can easily become infected to form a red and tender area. It will resist healing until the ingrown hair is freed. To do this it is necessary to nick the overgrown surface layer of skin and uncoil or completely remove the hair shaft with a pair of tweezers.

Many men suffer from ingrown hairs of the neck, regardless of the shaving method they use. The architecture of some of the hair follicles in this area are such as to promote the roofing over of skin when the hair is shaved off. Freeing such hairs from time to time is of limited and immediate benefit only, since the routine of shaving perpetuates the problem. Some men are rarely spared from tender, red, unpleasant-looking bumps scattered about the bearded area of the neck.

In my experience, I have found the best solution to this problem has been the permanent removal of these scattered troublesome hairs by electrolysis. After the ingrown hair has been freed, the operator (electrologist) destroys the hair in the usual fashion. Since this hair can never regrow, the problem for that follicle is ended. All the hairs of the neck are not involved; only those that create the difficulty are removed. With a little patience and persistence complete freedom from such ingrown hairs is accomplished without noticeable loss of the bearded portion of the neck.

The Loss of Scalp Hair

As mentioned in a previous section, a certain amount of hair is normally shed each day by men and women. Such hairs are in a normal resting phase from growth. While this may be as many as one hundred hairs daily, you may never be conscious of any diminution in scalp hair because there is a constant replacement by the hairs that are continually entering a growing cycle.

Of course, with aging, fewer hairs re-enter the growth cycle, and therefore older people show general thinning of scalp hair. This is more apparent in men than in women. There are several other causes for permanent hair loss. These may be related to specific, but not common, scarring skin diseases that may affect the scalp or a few general systemic diseases that affect hair growth (such as thyroid disease). These conditions cannot be considered in this book.

In my experience there are five common types of hair loss problems, including male pattern baldness which should be discussed here. Hair loss, of any type, always causes much concern. It is reason enough to consult your physician for a proper evaluation of your problem. Well-meaning beauty salon operators or barbers are not qualified to provide you with a learned opinion. Avoid the commercial hair and scalp clinics that promote hair growing methods. Seek the advice of medical experts. The discussion that follows is not a substitute for such advice.

BROKEN-OFF HAIR FROM SIMPLE HAIR DAMAGE. There is no injury to the growing portion of the hair. The hair shafts themselves break off because of the excessive use of chemicals and/or the combined physical effects that result from bleaching, toning, waving, straightening, teasing or other manipulation. Casual examination of such hair will immediately reveal varying lengths of the shafts. *The hair will always regrow.* You need only be patient, practice increased gentleness in caring for your hair, as described elsewhere, and avoid or postpone procedures that are known to influence hair shaft structure. If the breakage is extreme so that a satisfactory coiffure is not possible, a wig or fall will easily tide one over the period necessary for normal regrowth to occur.

COIN-SHAPED PATCHES OF BALDNESS. These appear on the scalp, suddenly, in both men and women and are known as *alopecia areata*. The cause for these perfectly clear patches is unknown, although there are many fascinating theories. Frightening to behold, they are usually of little consequence. The lost hair will, with only rare exception, always regrow—often without any treatment. The only time for concern, and this is quite unusual, is if new patches appear before old ones have regrown and areas appear to be blending with each other to produce larger zones of baldness. At such times your physician will institute a program of treatment to promote hair growth.

HAIR LOSS AFTER CHILDBIRTH. This is probably only an apparent hair loss rather than a real loss. The usual alternating cycles of growth and rest of the scalp hair are not followed for the duration of the pregnancy. Few, if any, hairs enter the resting phase. Following delivery of your child, the normal growth and rest cycles return. However, during this post-delivery period of adjustment, many more hairs than usual loosen and fall as the normal process catches up with itself.

No treatment is necessary. An understanding of the reason for the fall is enough to satisfy most women. In a few months, normalcy returns. Recently the Swedish and British medical literature has described temporary hair loss associated with a deficiency in the body stores of iron. Anemia itself need not be present, but blood loss associated with childbirth or excessive blood donations could be a factor. Such hair loss may respond to the administration of iron under medical supervision.

THINNING HAIR IN YOUNG WOMEN. In recent years all dermatologists have been seeing an increasing number of women with complaints of definite uniform thinning of hair over the mid-frontal portions of the scalp. The exact cause is not known; careful medical work-up has failed to reveal any basis for the hair loss, although several interesting leads have been uncovered. Perhaps the iron deficiency recently described in Swedish and British publications mentioned above may be a factor.

Since this type of hair loss is a new phenomenon observed in an era where there is a marked increase in frequency and severity of hair manipulation (use of tight rolling, nightly pin-ups, elaborate hair styling procedures, etc.) to satisfy fashion requirements, it is convenient to associate the two.

In my opinion there is some justification for this association. Many of my patients with this type of hair loss have shown an improvement after following a revised and simplified program for hair care and styling. It is most important to remember that patience is required. Hair, when it is growing, does so at about ½–¾ inch per month. It takes about a year to grow six to nine inches of hair—enough to comb and style. Often the hair follicles of the scalp where the thinning has taken place are in a resting or non-growing phase. It may take one or more months of waiting just for such hair bulbs to enter a growing phase. Unfortunately, everyone is in too much of a hurry for results—particularly the afflicted one.

If you have noticed thinning of the frontal portions of your scalp and have made the decision to reduce hair manipulation and change your coiffure to a simple one requiring little care, you will examine your scalp daily, hoping to find luxuriant regrowth from one day to the next. You will not find it. Benefit will only be found from one season to the next. This is a normal limitation—a fact of life which, however frustrating it is, cannot be changed. If your hair loss has been extreme, wigs or falls are excellent means for improving appearance during the months required for your hair to regrow.

MALE PATTERN BALDNESS. This progressive hair loss, which is predetermined by heredity, may begin in the teens (premature male pattern baldness) or at any time in life and proceed at its own individual rate of speed. The rate at which hair is lost in succeeding years need not be constant; therefore it is not possible for anyone to predict your hair status in the future.

At the present time, for this type of baldness, there is no practical or safe medication, method, procedure or combination of these that is known either to retard hair loss or to promote genuine hair growth in its affected follicles. I make this categoric statement early in this discussion so that you will know my position without having to search for it. Any claim that is made to the contrary, regardless of its source or expansiveness, and regardless of any photographs purporting to document improvement, is not referring to male pattern baldness or is merely referring to a medical curiosity without practical significance.

This does not mean that there will never be a practical or safe answer to this problem. However, should one be found, I feel certain it will be the culmination of good, reliable, past, present, and future scientific investigative labors rather than the chance discovery of a talented composer of concoctions, incantations, or devices.

Men of all ages, particularly the young—even boys accompanied by their mothers—are seen almost daily by me, and every other dermatologist, in the search for what can be done to stop or prevent the obvious progression of male pattern baldness.

Other than offering a reasonable explanation of the problem, a sincere attempt to help you adjust to the inevitable, and some few suggestions on controlling dandruff and care of your scalp as mentioned previously—gentle infrequent shampoos, patting dry (no rubbing) with a towel, combing and brushing lightly—nothing can be done.

In many individuals adjustment to the balding tendency comes slowly, reluctantly, and only after much time and money and hope have been left in hair parlors whose very survival depends on such human weaknesses.

For those who cannot ever adjust to this hair loss, or for those whose livelihood is closely linked with a personal appearance that demands a full head of hair, or for those men who just wish to improve their appearance, it is strongly recommended that they wear a hairpiece.

Toupees, as with all hand-crafted items, are available in many qualities. The more realistic and serviceable the hairpiece, the greater the skill and craftsmanship that is required to produce it. Prices range from less than $100 to more than $1000. Many men have found great comfort and satisfaction from their use. It requires some personal drive to overcome the initial resistance to the concept. This resistance has its origin outside the individual. If there were no friends, neighbors or associates to scrutinize the toupee, its initial wearing would offer no more problem than putting on a hat. Once the friends and associates have been broken in, it's free and easy living from then on.

The disadvantages are few. Depending upon the quality and style of your hairpiece, there will be limitations on its wearability under specific situations, particularly in certain sports. Several times each year the hairpiece must be cleaned and refurbished by experts to maintain its good appearance. This expense can be more than $100 per year, depending upon its craftsmanship.

There is an interesting new approach to the balding problem known as hair weaving. Luxuriant commercial human hair can be added to your own to produce a very natural and attractive appearance. It can be successfully performed only on heads that have some hair on the crown, even though sparse.

The operator weaves a strong lattice of nylon filaments into which the sparse scalp hair itself is incorporated. The nylon lattice is therefore "permanently" and quite rigidly fixed to your scalp. The lattice is skillfully shaped and placed in a predetermined position based on the amount of commercial hair to be used and the manner in which it is to be styled. The commercial hair is human hair that is matched to your own for color and texture. Unless great care is taken in this matching and blending stage, the end result will be disappointingly artificial. The hair mass is then attached by a weaving process to the lattice foundation. It is then cut, thinned, and shaped to blend with your natural hair and head contour, following which it is styled and combed as desired. The entire procedure can be carried out in one visit of three to four hours' time. Because the lattice foundation was carefully planned in advance, your hair, natural and added commercial, can be parted in its styling to reveal only natural scalp! This has great cosmetic importance.

Your new hair will not fall off nor can you take it off. It can be removed only by unweaving. Consequently, there are few limitations placed on your normal activities, regardless of their severity. You comb and shampoo your hair in the conventional manner. Any barber can be instructed merely to trim the sides of your naturally growing hair; he must leave the added hair untouched. Since hair grows at about ½–¾ inch per month, within three or four months the lattice, which was originally closely applied to your scalp, has loosened. Consequently, it is necessary to return to the operator three to six times per year to have the weave tightened.

Hair weaving requires expert craftsmanship to produce successful and satisfying results. Unfortunately, increasing popularity of the method has attracted a number of hastily or poorly trained operators interested primarily in quick financial gain rather than reliable workmanship and service.

The initial cost of hair weaving is approximately $400, with annual maintenance at about $120 per year. This is probably no more expensive than a good toupee. Except for a sensation of tightness over the scalp for a day or two following the procedure, little discomfort is experienced. However, it is an interesting new approach to a very troublesome problem.

No discussion of the subject could be complete without consideration of the surgical method for correcting baldness. It is known as the *hair transplant*. Most balding men are not completely hairless over the scalp. A reasonably dense fringe at the sides remains to frame the sparse or completely bald crown and frontal scalp. The principle of this surgical method is to transplant hair from the fringe area to the "top" of the head.

This is a minor and easily tolerated surgical operation that can be, and usually is, performed in the dermatologist's or surgeon's office following the local injection of anaesthetic. The procedure is as follows: After anaesthetizing the areas of the scalp to be treated, a sharp round instrument known as a "punch" is used to remove a plug of skin less than ½ inch in diameter from a hairless portion of your scalp. An exactly similar plug of skin is removed from the hairy fringe and placed as a graft in the first punched-out site. It is allowed to grow in this new transplanted area. The hairless plug of skin is discarded as useless; the hole in the fringe area left by the transplanted plug of hair quickly heals by itself. Usually twenty-five plugs of hairy tissue are transplanted at each treatment. The operator carefully positions the plugs over the frontal and uppermost portions of the scalp to tailor a new hairline. It takes approximately three months for your transplanted skin to grow its tuft of hair in its new location.

Every week or two, depending on your tolerance and urgency, twenty-five plugs are transplanted until approximately three hundred have been accomplished. Except for mild tenderness over the healing treated sites, there is little physical discomfort. The donor sites soon heal with a scar that is hairless. However, these are well hidden by the surrounding hair growth from this fringe portion of the scalp.

There is no doubt that this method has successfully and permanently transplanted actively growing hairs to balding areas of the scalp. Many patients have been satisfied with the results. If each tuft grows ten hairs (a rather liberal estimate), then three thousand hairs have been placed in a cosmetically valuable area of your scalp—the hairline and frontal scalp regions. These hairs, when long, can cover, to some extent, the previously bald regions of your scalp. To the man whose goal was to get some hair growing, there is significant satisfaction. Unfortunately, too many men are searching for new, thick, luxuriant growth. Such patients remain dissatisfied.

Since the treatments are usually performed on a Friday, with the weekend for recovery from the mild effects of the surgery, you need lose no time from your employment. There are many dermatalogists and surgeons who are performing this procedure throughout the world. The cost per treatment will vary and may be $100 or more per session for twelve sessions.

It is interesting to speculate on what might be accomplished if the hair transplant operation were combined with the hair-weaving technique. The latter requires some hair upon which to anchor and build its foundation lattice. That is why it cannot be used on a completely bald surface. Perhaps one could transplant a few hundred hairs to strategic areas of the scalp. These could then be used by the hair weaver for his lattice. Luxuriant commercial hair could then be fixed in place. If successful, this would satisfy another large group of men who have found the transplant method alone rather unsatisfactory.

NAIL CARE XII

Within the limitations of inherited qualities, personal habits and occupational hazard, some basic principles, practices, and products will help achieve attractive nails.

The nailplate is derived from epidermal cells of the skin. Its chemical make-up, despite the unique physical form and texture, is very similar to the keratin protein of the outer layer of the skin and the hair shaft.

You learn to depend on your fingernails to perform special tasks, such as picking up coins from flat surfaces, and using them as cutters, scrapers or wedges to pry things open. The presence of the nails is not always necessary; within a few minutes' re-education, you can learn to perform most little tasks as efficiently and far more safely with substitute aids.

As with hair, the nails, properly cared for, significantly improve your personal appearance. Long fingernails are particularly attractive because they give the impression of thin, tapered and graceful fingers. As fingernails become too long they actually reduce the efficiency of the hand's performance. They become an obstruction.

There are normal variations in the physical appearance and qualities of nailplates from person to person, and even from finger to finger in some individuals. These differences are caused by inherited characteristics plus the past or present history of a particular nail. Some people grow thicker, harder nails just as some grow heavier and coarser hair. Some nail plates possess vertical ridges because they are actually formed in this manner by exactly comparable distortions in the nail bed.

You must be constantly aware that your nails are also affected by their environment. Chemicals in industry, in hobbies or in the household, such as solvents, soaps, detergents, waxes, polishes, paints, varnishes, adhesives, cleaning fluids, bleaches, dyes, petroleum products and hundreds more, affect the nail plate just as they do the skin. But the skin sheds, replaces itself rapidly—total turnover in about twenty-six days. The uppermost portion of the epidermis, the keratin, is replaced every thirteen to fourteen days. Consequently, repeated chemical exposure of minor severity may produce no noticeable alterations in the skin of the hands because of the relatively rapid skin-cell turnover. The skin keratin just isn't around long enough to show the effects. However, it takes about six months for your fingernails to replace themselves completely. This is a very slow turnover rate. The nail plates are around a long time. They are exposed to repeated minor chemical action, called hydrolysis, to produce in some instances brittleness, flaking, splitting, chipping, and discoloration of the nail keratin— even separation of the plate from its bed in some instances.

Nail plates can easily be physically worn

down as a normal event during many hand tasks. Common, routine household chores often are particularly damaging. For example, while dishwashing itself exerts chemical effects upon the nailplates, scouring a pot or pan with a ball of steel wool actually grinds down the nailplate as effectively as if it had been clipped off. Grabbing a handful of salt from a bowl while cooking, sorting silverware from a pile, and many other operations are equally wearing.

Some occupations, to susceptible individuals, are notorious for their effects upon the nail and its surrounding tissue. These jobs require the hands to be wet for long periods of time; housekeepers, launderers, cooks, bartenders, food-handlers (particularly salad makers), dishwashers, etc. Red, tender, swollen areas of one or more fingers may appear about the skin fold that surrounds the nail plate; at times, pus may drain. There may be throbbing pain. The household word for such infections is "whitlow," and they require the attention of a physician.

Bear in mind that there are many diseases that can affect the nails to produce thickening, discoloration, peeling, splitting, separation, and even shedding. These may be such common skin diseases as psoriasis or various fungous infections, or systemic diseases such as anemia and thyroid conditions.

It is beyond the scope of this book to discuss nail problems that result from disease processes. Our interest is in the nail problems that result from common, ordinary, everyday abuse that can be corrected by good nail hygiene. With a little care and ambition, it is possible to acquire attractive nails. Don't pay attention to your nails only when some special event is approaching, at which time you expect the local cosmetic counter salesgirl or a manicurist to conjure up a miracle from within her many prettily colored bottles. A few coats of nail enamel may cover much you'd like to hide. However, nail enamel does more than camouflage. It dresses nails to emphasize their beauty and grace.

To accomplish anything with nails, you have to have them first. Unlike neglected hair, which can be made beautiful within hours, neglected nails may have insufficient nailplate available with which to work. You can begin to improve your nails as you read these lines. Reflect for a moment on your personal habits. If you pick at, or bite, your cuticles or nails, you are inflicting much damage to them. One way of successfully smashing this habit is to begin a manicure routine. If this hasn't helped you in the past, try diverting the picking reflex with harmless fidgeting in the form of doodling or playing with "worry beads." A long-chained, smooth-surfaced locket is great for fingering. Any replacement like this will spare your nails.

You must allow the nail and its surrounding structures to grow so that they can be properly groomed and shaped. Pay particular attention to the way you use and abuse your nails during the course of a busy day. How much are they subjected to a wearing-down process or a manipulation that simply breaks off nails? If you "think nails" throughout the day you can easily find ways to protect them from ordinary and steady wear and tear.

Never dial a telephone with a fingertip; use a pencil instead. Avoid the grasping maneuver when it means your fingertips will strike a hard surface, as a table top. Most objects can be picked up by trapping them between the straightened fingers. Then as you bring your fingers together the object is held quite firmly by the sides of the fingers (see SKETCHES 12–1 a and b). Other objects, like coins, can be swept into your other hand from a table top or can be picked up with a stiff piece of paper, such as a calling card. Do not acquire purses, wallets, key cases, etc. that require wear on nails to pry them open. The latch or clasp on any object should be replaced or completely avoided if it is a hazard to your nails or if its design defies substitute methods of operation. Letters and packages are easily opened with a sharp instrument other than a fingernail.

Many tasks can be easily performed with the ball of the finger as the finger is held in a straightened (extended) position. In this way

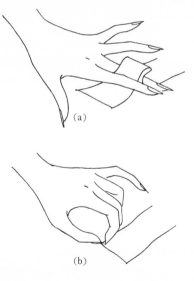

SKETCH 12–1: *Nail wear can be reduced and damage avoided by learning to spare the nails from unnecessary injury. For example, remember to pick up objects as illustrated in (a). The common method, as shown in (b) leads to splitting, chipping and erosion of the nail plates which strike the table top and each other.*

the nailplate itself is spared from friction and sudden shocks. I have known many good typists who type in this manner. I have also known musicians, even pianists, who worked out a compromise method of holding the fingers to spare their fingernails.

Handles have been added to all aids for keeping house, including dishwashing and pot scouring. Protective gloves should be handy at all vital centers of the house and worn for the many jobs that can injure nails and irritate skin.

Of course a regular, weekly, professional manicure to someone who is practicing daily fingernail protection will produce attractive nails. You can accomplish similar results, at home, if you will follow my suggested regimen. Remember that it takes months to grow a new nailplate—one whose basic chemistry has not been badly damaged by long-term physical insult. Therefore, don't get discouraged; you must have patience and diligence.

Nail Enamel Remover

If you are wearing nail enamel, remove it as follows: Saturate a cotton ball with the remover and quickly rub it over the nailplates of one hand to remove the great bulk of the old enamel; follow rapidly, where necessary, with a clean dry tissue to further improve removal. Any remnants of old enamel at the sides of the nail plate or near the skin fold should be taken off with a cotton-tipped applicator stick that is moist with remover. Do not attempt to do this with the cotton ball. Do not dip the fingertip directly into the remover.

Nail enamel removers are efficient solvents designed to do a special job. Their action should be confined to the nail plate alone for just the time required to get rid of old enamel. Some products are faster acting than others; some contain oils to prevent the old dissolved enamel from staining the fingers that are holding the cotton ball (non-smudge type). Other differences exist in the quality of the solvent itself and the fragrance added to minimize the pungent odor characteristic for such solvents, thereby making their use more pleasant. Begin the second hand when you have completed the process on the first.

An emery board for shaping the nail is preferred since it is more flexible than the standard metal file. However, the new type, emery-like metal files are excellent. Do not use the sharp point for ambitious digging under and around nails where injury may possibly result. File down any loose or ragged edges of the nail tip by filing from each side of the nail plate toward its center. Avoid back and forth sawing movements by stroking in one direction only. The goal is to achieve an oval-shaped nail.

Filing

Never file into the extreme corners of the nail—the zone where the nail plate edge meets the sides of the fingertip (see SKETCH 12–2). This is a valuable, strong natural nail edge which must grow out *intact*. To file into this corner is like fraying the hem of a dress. In addition, weakening this corner promotes the formation of the often painful hangnail.

It is not advisable to cut or clip nail plates since this produces a shearing action on the nail plate that weakens its natural structure and promotes fracturing and splitting.

Cuticle Care Immersing the fingers for three or more minutes in a bath of warm, slightly soapy water cleanses the nailplates, the skin about the nails, and softens the cuticle—the fold of skin at the nail plate edge which joins with the finger itself (see SKETCH 2–8c, p. 27). The solution your manicurist uses is more efficient than soap. Special solutions for aiding you in this procedure at home are available, if you prefer. This is a simple step during a professional manicure for one hand soaks while the manicurist is busy with the other. In the self-manicure this becomes a chore and cuticle softening is usually left to the product known as *cuticle remover*. When time and patience permit, the finger soak is worth taking. Dry the fingertip and gently remove any soil in the crevices about and under the nail. This can be done with the blunted tip of a wooden or plastic orange stick.

As new nail is formed and grows outward, the skin fold (cuticle), particularly at the base where the "moon" or lighter-colored nail is apparent, tends to adhere to the plate. For the most attractive, oval-shaped nails, it is necessary to retract this portion of the cuticle. *Gently*

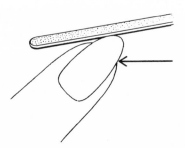

SKETCH 12–2: *Shape your nails to a graceful oval. File from each side of the nail plate toward its center. Be sure to* avoid *the extreme corner on each side as illustrated by the arrow and emery board in this illustration.*

push back the softened cuticle from the plate itself in the region of the moon with the flat end of the orange stick.

Occasionally, not necessarily at each manicure, it is recommended that a cuticle remover cream be applied to the cuticle area only and permitted to remain in place for five to ten minutes, or as directed by the manufacturer. This easy-to-use product actually softens the tissues to make pushing back the cuticle from the nail a much easier operation. After the specified time has elapsed, rinse off the cuticle softening cream thoroughly in fresh running water; dry the fingers and *gently* push back the cuticle from the nailplate with the orange stick so that a clean and full nailplate will gradually develop. *Do not attempt to accomplish too much.*

This must be a slow and careful procedure. It will take weeks of cuticle training to push it back far enough to achieve a bigger moon area and a flattering oval shape to the nail plate. You must not be too vigorous in your pushing. You are actually separating the fold of skin from a portion of the nail plate where the skin is not needed. If you try to do too much at one time, you can deliberately injure the nail plate or the nail bed itself. This may cause eventual ridging of your nail. For this reason the novice is better off using a wooden or plastic stick rather than one made of metal.

It is not necessary to use the stick at each manicure. This is particularly important once you have shaped the cuticle fold well and have a graceful moon at the nail base. You can easily maintain this shape by blunt pressure. To do this, place a soft towel over your right thumb and grasp a fingertip of the left hand between it and your right index finger. The toweled thumb pad must be pressing firmly against the fingernail. Push the cuticle back; the towel allows good contact to move the cuticle. Do each finger in turn. Then switch the towel to your left thumb and do the same to the cuticle areas of your right hand.

The cuticle remover is so named because its mission is to help in releasing the cuticle from its firm attachment to the new nail plate. It will also clean off any remnants of skin that adhere to the nail so that the plate itself will have a smooth, even surface. It is not expected that the cuticle tissue itself should be removed from the finger. *The band of cuticle must stay!* As with all skin, it sheds itself gradually and imperceptibly; and it replaces itself. You should not cut the cuticle. If a loose edge appears, it may be carefully clipped off; but do not attempt to trim off the entire semicircular cuticle rim. It is very tempting to do this and it appears to be a common practice. However, better overall results will be achieved if this firm band of protective skin is left intact.

Nail Enamel Application

At this time it is wise to gently scrub your nails with a nail brush and warm soapy water to remove any soil or debris that may have gathered in the crevices about the nail. As you dry your hands, use the towel folded over your thumb to give the cuticles another gentle push. Then examine the nails carefully for any final grooming before proceeding with the application of enamel.

For best results, the application of nail enamel must follow the same principles that have been practiced for centuries by enamel and lacquer craftsmen.

1. The surface must be clean and free of soaps and oils.
2. When necessary a prime or base coat material should be applied.
3. Apply a fresh, quality enamel with a single, quick, definite stroke. Do not stroke over again.
4. Thin applications are better than thick ones.
5. Each coat must dry thoroughly before another is applied.
6. Several properly applied coats will look better and outwear fewer but heavier layers.

First check the shade of enamel you intend to wear. Shake the bottle well to mix its contents. This must be done even to enamel that has just been purchased. If previously used, open the vial and make sure that it flows freely from its brush; if it is too thick do not use it. Adding nail enamel remover as a thinner will not salvage the product. It is a waste of effort to work with such material and the end result is never satisfying.

Sit comfortably at a well-lighted table. The fingers to be enameled should rest on the rigid table top—not suspended in air nor held in the lap. The enamel bottle must be conveniently placed nearby. You will find it more comfortable to use a long-handled brush that can be held much like a pencil. Therefore, screw the wand some manufacturers provide into the cap of the bottle.

Clean the nail surface once more with nail enamel remover. Each nail can be coated with three, deliberate, full-length strokes of the brush; one down the center of the nail and one down each side (see SKETCH 12–3). The brush should be redipped for each nail. Rebrushing over wet enamel will only distort the surface. If your first strokes do not seem to have covered the nail completely, all will be easily corrected with the next coat. Be sure to let each application dry thoroughly. If you apply two to three thin coats in this fashion you will achieve the best and longest-lasting coverage possible. Proceed to do all nails in rotation. The key to success is the use of a quality product. It will assure ease of application and improved wearability as well as the most attractive appearance. Do not leave the enamel bottle open unnecessarily. Be sure to wipe clean the mouth of the bottle before screwing down the cap. This will insure easy opening for the next manicure.

Some nail enamels will adhere better if a prime or base coat is applied to the nail (but be sure it dries thoroughly) before the enamel. For a glossier finish and improved wearability, a special top coat is available.

It is absolutely necessary that you get, or give yourself, a manicure regularly, usually at weekly intervals. Only in this manner, in con-

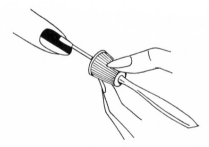

SKETCH 12–3: *Nail enamel should be applied with deliberate, full-length strokes; one down the center of the nail, and one down each side. Thin coats are best; do not rebrush while wet. The second and third coats will provide complete and even coverage.*

junction with practicing nail protection and sparing, will you be able to acquire attractive nails.

There are other good nail procedures that also encourage the development of attractive nails. For the most part they require significant additional attention and some variation in the manicuring routine.

Nail Buffing

After the nails have been shaped and the cuticles adequately cared for, as described above, a small amount of buffing cream is applied and allowed to dry on the nails. Then stroke repeatedly across the nailplate with a suitable buffing pad or chamois cloth to produce a luster.

This is an attractive finish when nail enamel is not going to be used. While it may not satisfy the demands of the fashion-conscious woman, it is quite acceptable for many occasions. (Most manicures for men are finished in this manner.) It is certainly more attractive than enamel that shows signs of wear.

There appears to be some advantage in nail care hygiene if you divide the manicure routine into sessions. This is especially true for the person who has nails that tend to flake, split or break off easily. For example, remove your enamel in mid-week and follow through with filing and cuticle care. Then buff your nails for the next day or two. As the busy week-end approaches, you need only spend time in the careful application of the proper shade of enamel. Since buffing creams contain waxes, it is imperative that the nails be thoroughly cleansed with enamel remover before your enamel is applied.

An evening or two during the week, if nail

enamel is not worn, avail yourself of the opportunity for lubricating your nails with any of the nail creams or oils that are available to help counteract flaking, peeling or splitting.

Mention should be made at this time of other special nail products that are available.

Hardeners and Conditioners

It is logical to assume that if the nail substance itself could be influenced, it might be possible to improve the wearability or "hardness" of the nailplate. Theoretically, the greatest influence on nail substance will occur at its point of production—deep in the nail bed. In addition to injury, infection, and local disease, it is known that poor nutrition, poor circulation, anemia, thyroid disease and other internal problems can serve seriously to affect the quality of your nail substance. It has been rather popular belief, even among some physicians, that an increase in the body intake of protein might aid in the production of a better nail. An easy way to add protein to the diet is by eating gelatin. Of course, this would only influence the new nail that is being made; it would take months of continuous ingestion before any benefit could be observed in nail texture.

A person who is poorly nourished, or who suffers because of a low protein diet, may benefit from stepped-up protein intake. Swallowing gelatin capsules or a tablespoonful of gelatin dissolved in fruit juice (at room temperature) two or three times daily may indeed, after six months, yield an improved nail. The patients who enter my office with complaints of soft, flaking and fragile nails exhibit no evidence of protein deficiency. In the few trial instances where gelatin was added to their daily diet it succeeded only in increasing their body weight.

Protein (which is what the nail is essentially made of) can be hardened by certain chemicals which are also known as tissue fixatives. One of the best of such fixatives is formaldehyde. Formaldehyde-type nail hardeners—dilute solutions for painting on the nail substance itself— have been available and used with some success. Such products may have a greater potential for producing allergic skin reactions than the public has learned to expect from cosmetics. In addition, their misuse for nail conditions other than to promote nailplate hardness has made them unpopular items on the cosmetic counter. Some of my colleagues in dermatology, impressed with the hardening ability of formaldehyde, have advised me that they have had to resort to writing prescriptions to duplicate such products for their patients.

Another group of nail hardening preparations functions merely to temporarily support the fragile, flaking and splitting nail by coating it with a strong film, quite similar to a clear nail enamel. In some instances, nylon fibers are suspended in the thick liquid so that on application to the nail, the dried film with fibers enmeshed provides greater strength. These film-formers are designed to be worn alone or under nail enamel. Unfortunately, the irregular surface of the dry film reduces the cosmetic elegance of any nail enamel that is applied to it.

Several products are available with the name nail conditioner that are known to contain protein-type substances. These are painted on the bare nail for strengthening the plate. As with hair conditioners such preparations serve to fill in tiny imperfections in the nailplate itself to offer a degree of improved nailplate quality. Such products, of course, can not influence the growth pattern or characteristics of the nail itself. Although nail enamel may be applied over these conditioners, the wearability of the enamel may, in some instances, be reduced.

The Nail Patch Accidents do happen to modestly long and very long nailplates even though you have been most diligent in observing good nail habits. A partial break or split, if not too extensive, can be mended to preserve the plate for a considerable period of time. The repair is often accomplished without major sacrifice in appearance. It is well worth the effort.

Although convenient nail-fixing kits can be found where you purchase your nail enamel, the materials needed are simple and often readily at hand: absorbent cotton or facial tissue and a clear nail enamel or base coat.

Remove the nail enamel and cleanse the damaged plate carefully. Saturate a patch of

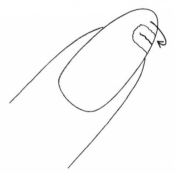

SKETCH 12–4: *A nail patch can often successfully mend a split nail plate to preserve its length and appearance. The patch should be wider than the split and cover both surfaces of the nail plate as illustrated.*

facial tissue, or a portion of shredded absorbent cotton, with the nail fixing fluid, base coat fluid or clear nail enamel; fold the patch over the split portion of the nail. The fold should be made so that the patch covers over the split on its upper as well as under nail surface (see SKETCH 12–4). It is possible to smooth down the patch snugly before it dries. Serious breaks may require a second layer.

The entire plate should now be covered with a few coats of base coat followed by nail enamel in the usual manner. While the repaired nail will now have a ridge in it that is created by the patch material, you have been able to preserve uniformity in nail length. The repair patch will require careful replacement with each manicure; eventually, as the nail grows out, the damaged portion is filed off.

The Artificial Nail

It is possible to purchase preformed plastic nails which are packaged in several shapes and sizes to conform to the normal nailplate configuration. The artificial nail is trimmed to fit the fingertip and affixed with a special adhesive supplied with the kit.

You must have some natural nail plate surface present to which the artificial nail can adhere. Badly ridged and thickened nailplates (as result from certain disease processes) do not accept the artificial nail very well. Consequently, the usefulness of artificial nails is considerably limited. In addition, it is quite time-consuming to apply properly to more than a finger or two.

Moisture, vibration, and the numerous daily shocks to the nails cause the artificial nail to loosen. It is best that they be removed after one or two days' wear anyway since constant application is not healthy. The adhesive material may cause considerable local tissue reaction in some users since its potential for producing allergy is significantly greater than that of most consumer products.

Somewhat similar to the above is the kit which permits the "building" of a plastic nail directly on the fingertip. A mold is fixed to the finger in the shape of a nail and the freshly mixed chemicals are added to the mold. When dry the mold form is removed and the artificial nail is then filed, shaped and enameled. This process has all the deficiencies of the preformed artificial nail. However, its ability to cause tissue reaction is even greater.

These products do have some value, particularly for individuals in the public eye. If one or two nails must be applied or "built up" to maintain uniform nail length for a specific event of short duration, then these kits can be very helpful.

The concept of the artificial nail is intriguing; it is the source of much investigation. New compounds are constantly being developed and investigated. The possibility for creating rigid plastics and adhesives that possess excellent compatibility with living tissue is very good in the immediate future.

Good nail hygiene and grooming contribute much to your appearance. It is well worth the effort, for your nails complement your hands which are constantly in view. They serve as a means of expression. They greet friends and acquaintances, emphasize points of conversation, and even contribute to your departure in the final gesture of a good-bye wave.

Nail products used regularly and wisely can

give you much help. They are beauty and grooming aids only. Remember that nails are merely extensions of your skin and are subject to disease processes. The nail products and routines described in this chapter cannot remove inherited nail weaknesses nor treat nail diseases such as psoriasis, fungous infections, and paronychia. But they can help you to overcome the nail problems that result from daily abuse. Nail biters, housewives, career girls, businessmen can all become proud of their nails.

XIII SUNDRY ITEMS OF
SUBSTANCE AND CONSEQUENCE

Good overall skin care includes an understanding of the special problems of foot and leg hygiene, and of the effect of exercise, massage, heat and rest.

Foot Care The dictates of custom and fashion are particularly demanding to our feet. During waking hours they are usually confined in footgear that often is too restrictive; ventilation and light are poor or non-existent. As upright, biped creatures, no portion of our body suffers more from circulatory problems than the legs and feet. While blood may travel to them with ease, its equally important return trip must work against the pull of gravity. This return circulation to the heart is necessary for the removal of waste products and the replenishment of supplies for tissue requirements. Blood that stagnates will soon cause serious problems.

Many occupations, including household chores, require the legs to remain in the dependent position (this includes sitting) for long periods of time. Muscular activity to help blood circulation is often of inadequate degree. During our leisure time, the same pattern of insult to the legs and feet is continued.

You rarely find or make opportunities to elevate your legs to help out your circulation. The need for this becomes greater as you get older. Tired, swollen feet and ankles at the end of the day, or varicose veins (prominent out-pocketing of veins of the legs) are frequently the more obvious signs of poor circulation in this part of your body.

Why is this a subject for a book on skin care? Because circulatory deficiencies have a serious effect on the skin of your legs and feet. Any injury to your legs or feet, however minor, will require a longer period of time to heal than is customary for injuries elsewhere. The skin of these freshly healed areas is usually darker in color, more pigmented than the surrounding skin. It may take many months for this discoloration to disappear.

With increasing deterioration in the return circulation, the skin about your lower legs may become itchy and show signs of a rash that does not seem to heal. An injury to such skin, as trifling as a bump against a table leg, may cause an open wound. It may heal with difficulty, or not at all. For such chronic leg ulcers you must seek the care of a physician for expert management. Not only can your skin be healed, but you will receive valuable advice for improving the circulation to your lower limbs. Where necessary, local medical treatment or surgical procedures may be carried out to correct the varicose veins.

Your feet and legs deserve a little special attention, therefore, to maintain better skin health and improved appearance. Cleanse daily with warm water—soap is not essential each time unless soil is present. As body oils and perspiration about your legs diminish, particularly after age thirty-five, excessive use of soap or detergents should be avoided. Learn to substitute a cleansing cream or lotion similar to those used for your face. A few products of this type have been particularly designed for the legs and feet. Their consistency and texture make application and removal easy and comfortable.

Be certain the skin between your toes is dried thoroughly after the bath or shower and then powdered to maintain as much freedom from moisture as possible. This will also reduce odor. Ordinary body dusting powder may be used or one of the many foot powders. Most foot powders contain antiseptic agents which provide better protection from the invasion of microscopic organisms such as fungi. Fungi are commonly present on the skin of the toes of most people. However, the fungi usually cause no problem until particular changes take place in their environment—changes which promote growth, multiplication and invasion. Warmth, moisture, and darkness is the environment that is most accommodating to fungi. Warmer weather or physical effort that causes your feet to perspire in footgear is ideal for developing the itching, peeling and discomfort of athlete's foot. Careful and frequent cleansing, thorough drying and dusting with foot powder will help you avoid athlete's foot.

In my experience, athlete's foot is rare in children under twelve years of age. The peeling and skin erosions that may occur about the toes in this younger age group are usually the result of excessive perspiration. At such times, it is most helpful to cleanse with little soap but much water; follow with careful drying and dusting with powder. If the problem continues, only socks of absorbent natural fiber should be worn, such as cotton in warm weather, wool in winter. Except in the most extreme instances, I have seen no reason to prefer white over colored socks.

Toenails grow at a slower rate than the fingernails. Do not permit them to extend much beyond the edge of your toes. Long toenails interfere with shoe comfort; under the pressure of walking the long nail will distort the natural position of your toes and may even cut into the skin of neighboring toes. Pain, swelling and infection occur which can be so disabling as to require medical, even surgical, attention.

Toenails should be clipped straight across their width. A portion or corner of nail must remain at the sides of each nailplate to cover the toe itself (see SKETCH 13–1).

If you attempt to clip the nail in a curve similar to that for fingernails, you will remove this valuable corner of nail. A real danger then exists of your developing an ingrown toenail. Ingrown toenails occur when the growing nail does not ride over the surface of the toe but

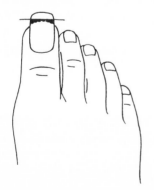

SKETCH 13–1: *Toenails should be clipped straight across their width in order to preserve the corners that can "ride" over the fleshy part of the toe edge. Attention to this detail will avoid painful ingrown toenails.*

begins to dig into the fleshy edge of the toe itself. The pressure created by shoes and the act of walking helps push the short-clipped nail into the skin fold of the toe. To avoid this serious problem, clip your toenails carefully. Be sure to preserve their corners so that they override the edges at the sides of the toe itself. A sharp, straight, heavy pair of scissors may be used to accomplish this. Toenail snippers are good only if they have straight blades. If your toenails are extremely thick, special instruments are necessary and the attention of a podiatrist is recommended. Gently file the clipped nail with an emery board to smooth each edge to prevent snags in hosiery.

If desired, the nailplate and cuticle may be groomed in a manner similar to that for the fingernails, including the application of nail enamel. If you are doing this yourself, be considerably more gentle than when caring for your fingernails; your toes are less accessible. You may tire easily. Be cautious to avoid any injury to these tissues which heal more slowly.

Corns and calluses are localized areas of extremely thickened keratin—the uppermost horny layer of the epidermis. This results from persistent friction or pressure upon a localized area, as from tight-fitting footwear, a pattern of walking, or the physical effort related to some sports activities.

The first danger signal of excessive friction or pressure is the appearance of a painful blister. The top layers of the skin are damaged by pressure and friction in a manner similar to a burn. If the cause of this tissue damage is not removed—if, for example, the offending shoes continue to be worn, then nature protects itself from further injury by producing the hardened skin—the corn or the callus. In this manner the skin can withstand future repeated injury without forming a blister and you will be spared discomfort.

In time, however, the constant pressure and friction will cause the corn or callus to become extremely thick and hard. Portions of it, particularly the center, will impinge upon sensitive nerves deep in the skin (dermis). Pressure upon the surface will cause pain which, at times, can be knife-like. You can obtain measurable relief by paring down the layers of dense, hard tissue. As the volume occupied by the corn or callus is reduced, there is a little more room in your shoe. Less pressure is exerted upon the nerve endings to minimize your distress.

Parings, however, do not cure your problem. As you persist in wearing the same or similar-type footgear, friction and pressure continues. Your skin, in its reaction to protect itself, keeps producing more hard keratin; the painful situation repeats itself.

Complete surgical removal of a corn or callus is also only a temporary measure as long as its basic cause remains, namely, improperly fitting footgear. A shoe may be the correct size and width for your foot, but a slightly misshapen toe that protrudes to cause friction or pressure will develop a corn. Such a shoe is still an improper fit. Most often, however, poorly fitting shoes are too short or too narrow. Toes are cramped and corns and calluses result.

Corns cannot be cured unless friction and pressure are removed *permanently*. This is difficult to accomplish once the corn has established itself—often many years after the first warning signs of redness, pain and blister formation have been forgotten.

This is not a plea for the wearing of sensible shoes. Fashion rarely means comfort. It is merely an attempt to explain a common problem. It is always easier to adjust to something you can understand. To help you adjust to your corns and calluses, periodic paring of the excess tissue is necessary. Razor blade paring should be reserved for the expert; it is very easy to injure yourself with such super-sharp instruments. The safest method is to soak your feet in warm water for ten to twenty minutes; damp-dry and rub the thickened callus or corn with a pumice stone or similar sandpaper-like device available at any drug counter. This will slowly but safely grind down the excess tissue. It may take several such treatments over a period of weeks to finally achieve adequate paring. Regular treatment in this manner will promote foot comfort.

The common wart is a firm growth of the upper layer of the skin that is caused by a skin virus. Susceptibility to this virus varies from person to person and this susceptibility can even change within an individual from time to time. The fingers are a common location for warts where they may appear in large number. Children seem particularly prone to warts although they can be found in any age group. Their appearance has nothing to do with handling toads.

The wart virus is quite common; and for reasons poorly understood it suddenly begins to grow in susceptible skin. Although an individual may infect other parts of his body (for example, a child who habitually bites the wart on his finger may finally infect the skin about his lips) the possibility for transmitting such common warts by casual contact with others is quite remote.

Warts on the fingers rarely produce pain; however, removal is usually sought because of their unattractiveness. Warts have responded to all forms of treatment; from Tom Sawyer's "spunk-water" as well as the most skilled technics of the physician-surgeon. Frustratingly, they have also defied every procedure, regardless of its sophistication. Final eradication of a wart may require infinite patience.

When this same wart virus grows on the weight-bearing surface of your foot—the sole (which is known as the plantar surface)—it is called a *plantar wart*. (This has nothing to do with tillers of the soil.) Because of the constant pressure of walking, the wart is forced to grow inward and may produce considerable pain with each step. Early treatment is desirable. Since such warts may be confused with a painful callus, the diagnosis must be made by the expert physician.

Tired, aching feet can adversely affect your personality and general well-being just as surely as a headache. Foot distress is often reflected in your face. With a little attention, it is possible to get lots more mileage out of your feet each day.

1. Cleanse your feet regularly and powder dry all surfaces.
2. Keep toenails just long enough to ride over all edges of the toes.
3. Pare down corns and calluses regularly with pumice stone.
4. Elevate feet whenever possible by resting them on a stool or similar object.
5. If fashion will not permit you to wear

roomy, comfortable and supportive foot-gear, then try to change shoes several times during the day.

6. Do not ignore a persistent foot problem. Seek out expert advice.

The appearance of the legs can be significantly improved by bleaching or removing the hair. This has been discussed elsewhere in this book. Routine application of lubricating emollients or moisturizing creams will aid in keeping the skin more soft and supple. Many specific leg make-up products are now available in several shades that can be worn alone or in combination with stockings. These products accomplish a more attractive and uniform appearance of the skin; their covering capacity significantly blends out minor skin discolorations. Apply this leg make-up with your hands in long sweeping strokes; it dries rapidly and withstands wear with insignificant rub-off. Removal is easily accomplished with soap and water or cleansing creams.

The Health Club Exercise, massage, and extremes of temperature cause stimulation or relaxation of physical and mental body functions. A feeling of well-being comes over you that may last for minutes or hours. With this contentment there follows an improvement in temperament that must be reflected in your personal appearance. You need only take a warm bath or shower to experience some of the benefits of this fundamental truth.

The steam room, the sauna and the massage table have been joined by a multitude of gadgets and devices which all serve a similar purpose— the promotion of active and passive exercise;

friction and mild irritation of the body surface; temperature and humidity variations. Regardless of their novelty or ingenious design they promote stimulation of body functions, some of which are not under voluntary control, such as sweating and dilation or constriction of blood vessels. As long as your body can tolerate exposure to this exertion, you will derive both physical and psychological benefit. If you have any doubt about your health, be sure to seek your physician's opinion in advance.

The skin, since it is most accessible, has always been subjected to manual measures such as pinching, slapping, stroking, friction and massage; nor has it been spared from attack by an infinite number of mechanical and electrical machines too numerous to mention. These may heat, cool, steam, rub, tap, etc. Others support, exercise or stimulate the "muscles." (There are no muscles in the skin worth stimulating. There are tiny evolutionary remnants associated with the hair follicles that cause "goose bumps" when you are chilled. These are the same type muscles which in an animal like the cat make its fur stand up when it is frightened.)

Cleverly devised variations of standard "health club" machines, encased in cabinets reflecting the space age motif, have been scaled down to accommodate the face and neck or isolated regions of the body. Although a few of these devices have been offered for home use, most of them are available only in well-appointed salons which cater to devotees who seek these routines and the special attention that accompanies them.

You may prefer or can afford to have others minister to your personal needs. Often this will provide good and reasonably expert routine care on a continuing basis that would otherwise be inconvenient or perhaps impossible for you to accomplish on your own. It is regular and repeated attendance which is the greatest advantage to any salon care. Regardless of the uniqueness of the mechanical or electrical devices involved, the personal attention promotes good skin hygiene, a pleasant sensation, and a feeling of accomplishment. If you disregard all other claims, stated or implied, made by the salon or its operators, these are sufficient reasons for embracing a salon program that suits you. You are certain to derive benefit from the supervision that hovers over you from visit to visit, keeping you interested and anxious to devote time and attention to your skin.

Regrettably, these simple reasons get buried in a kind of hocus-pocus and razzle dazzle. Some salon operators soon feel imbued with special skills and knowledge beyond that of mortal man. They become papier-mâché authorities—convincing on the outside but hollow within. Reasonable, intelligent, routine skin hygiene and care can be performed by anyone, at home or in a salon, with or without the aid of elaborate mechanical means. The secret to success is the interest in and the practice of a sensible routine. The stimulus from a salon is as good as from anywhere else. The very goal of this book is to stimulate you to become interested in caring for your skin.

The Effect of Rest

It is difficult if not impossible to feel sparkling, or to appear so, if you are physically exhausted. While good grooming and the clever application of make-up can and does lift your spirits as it improves your appearance, physical exhaustion will soon break through to reveal itself. You become inattentive and respond poorly to what is being said and to what is happening about you. Your eyes tend to droop and your facial expression becomes flat, depleted—coming alive momentarily only to suffer the distortion of a stifled yawn.

The beauty nap has often been a subject of humor. Napping will not make you beautiful; but lack of rest will most certainly keep you from looking your best, regardless of the effort and time you put into grooming, dressing and adorning yourself.

The average adult who enjoys reasonably good health requires no more than eight hours sleep per day. However, sleep requirements and habits vary widely from person to person. If you feel in need of more rest, a short nap before dressing for the evening will indeed be a beauty nap.

Some fortunate people have the ability to fall off to sleep almost anywhere, anytime, even under rather noisy and uncomfortable situations. Eye shields to block out light and ear stoppers to reduce noise level are handy gadgets that are available to aid in counteracting the common distractions that may keep you from sleeping. But even if sleep is not possible, reclining in a comfortable position and relaxing for thirty to sixty minutes is time well spent in the quest to look and feel your best.

The chin strap, often worn while napping, is purported to avoid or reduce skin sag or the double chin. In my opinion the only value to this appliance is that it may encourage you to take a nap.

Your Smile and Dental Care

Facial expression fortifies your physical appearance with charm. While eye movements send and receive messages, your mouth provides the real sparkle to your face. Your smile, no matter how modest and gentle, adds the glow of warmth, of life, to your personality. The mere hint of a frown can be repelling, cold, and austere.

The color and shape of your lips demand the care and attention described in the chapter on make-up. The attractive illusion you have created can be fortified by your exposed teeth or suddenly blurred, even shattered, by an open smile. You cannot afford to neglect the health and appearance of your teeth.

Daily, regular brushing, either by hand or by electric devices, the use of the newer pulsating streams of water for efficient cleansing of tooth crevices, and periodic professional attention are essentials for dental health. Your dentist, however, can do more than help you to keep and maintain sound teeth, or replace those which are beyond repair. He can assure you even, well-shaped, properly proportioned teeth.

Although efficient realignment of teeth, where necessary, is best accomplished in childhood, the adult can also benefit from *orthodontia*—the science and art of preventing and correcting irregularities in dental structure. Discolored or misshapen teeth are easily capped in natural white "jackets." If nature was not kind to you with regard to the shape of your exposed teeth (tooth structure and characteristics are inherited just as with any other physical trait), or if an unfortunate accident has chipped or broken a tooth vital to your appearance, seek the advice of your dentist. An attractive, sparkling smile can be yours.

Halitosis ("bad breath") refers to an unpleasant, offensive odor that may emanate from the mouth. Intimate contact, as in kissing, is not necessary to recognize halitosis. Often you can be aware of it while engaging in ordinary conversation.

Bad breath can be caused by many things. Its correction may require far more attention than a simple mouthwash or the chewing of a pleasantly scented confection.

Your breath normally has a slightly sweet odor. It will vary with age, becoming stronger as you get older. This odor also varies with the time of day; morning breath is strongest. The amount of saliva and the type of bacteria customarily present in your mouth will also influence the degree of normal odor.

Most offensive breath odors originate in the mouth. Tooth decay and diseases of the gums are common causes. Poor mouth hygiene encourages the decomposition of food remnants trapped about teeth and permits saliva to stagnate. Regular brushing of your teeth, mouthwashing, and periodic professional care can eliminate these causes.

Some breath odors, however, do not originate in the mouth. They are caused by the elimination of odors through the lungs—through the normal act of breathing. For example, the odor caused by foods and drink, such as onions, garlic, alcohol, and some medications, takes place in a very roundabout way. These odoriferous substances are absorbed from stomach and intestines into the bloodstream during digestion. The blood releases this odor into the lung air as it passes through the lung tissue. This lung air is then expired during normal breathing and the offensive odor becomes apparent. Brushing your teeth, washing out your mouth, or chewing a mint will only temporarily mask but not correct this type of odor. The elimination of such foodstuffs from your diet or substitution of the responsible medicaments is the only means of avoiding the offensive odor.

Diseases of the lungs and respiratory system, such as infections of lungs, sinuses, tonsils, or ordinary "post-nasal drip" may be responsible for halitosis. Your physician can help you correct these causes.

A reasonably simple way of determining whether breath odor is originating from your mouth or from structures of the respiratory system is the following: close your lips tightly; then breathe out forcefully through your nose. If someone else can smell an odor from this exhaled air, then the cause of the odor is probably from your respiratory system. If no odor is determined, then the cause, in all likelihood, originates from your mouth. Now pinch your nose closed with your fingers and exhale a soft, gentle breath of air from your mouth. If an odor is detected, it verifies that the cause of the halitosis is in your mouth.

The Accidental Ingestion of Cosmetics

Children, particularly toddlers, normally search out the new objects that come into their expanding world. Discoveries are, as a basic reflex, brought to the mouth to taste—and even to swallow—though they may not be particularly palatable.

Common household products, such as aspirin and laundry bleach, are frequently swallowed by children. Although cosmetics are not listed among the most frequently ingested household agents, on occasion they have been associated with such accidents.

Of course, the best and safest rule to follow is to keep all medications, cleaning and laundering materials, toiletries and cosmetics, etc. out of the reach of the roving and inquisitive child. Despite the security measures and vigilance in your own household, one day you may suddenly be confronted with accidental ingestion of an undesirable substance by either your child or a neighbor's child.

An emergency situation, particularly one such as this, can, with quick and intelligent action, be converted to a simple and routine problem. All it takes is a little advance preparation and knowledge. Every member of your family, the older children as well as the adults, should be familiar with the following rules for action when there has been ingestion of an undesirable substance.

Upon discovery, do not exhibit panic. Keep your wits, and above all, your temper. To raise your voice and to scold at this critical moment will result in the loss of vital information. Children are masters at interpreting your mood. If you convey panic and fear, if you become angry and scold the child, he will most certainly weep. The possibility, then, for getting reasonable cooperation from the child is destroyed.

If the child is old enough to talk, or only of the age to act out and jabber, he can be of considerable help in your getting a reasonable evaluation of the degree of hazard that has occurred. The child who is weeping and wailing compounds the confusion. Worst of all, this makes it difficult to determine whether he is crying now from fright, because of your scolding, or from pain or physical distress related to the material swallowed.

GENTLY, BUT FIRMLY, REMOVE THE BOTTLE, JAR, CAN, ETC. FROM THE CHILD'S POSSESSION. Even though the object is immediately recognized by you, it is extremely important to handle it with care for the information it will soon provide. Certainly your first thought is for the safety of the child. Simple and deliberate action will be to the child's benefit.

PLACE THE CONTAINER IN AN UPRIGHT POSITION WHERE IT WILL NOT BE ACCIDENTALLY KNOCKED OVER. Don't handle it with scorn or discard it in the waste basket.

SPEAK TO THE CHILD IN COMFORTING TONES while you blot up the substance that may be around his mouth and fingers.

GENTLY FLUSH THE MOUTH AND SURROUNDING SKIN with large amounts of fresh water. Then give him his bottle or a glass of milk to sip.

IF THE SUBSTANCE IS CLASSIFIED AS A HAZARDOUS SUBSTANCE by federal and local governments, the label will bear instructions for emergency care in the event of accidental ingestion.

TRY TO FIGURE OUT HOW MUCH THE CHILD MAY HAVE SWALLOWED by careful observation and some rough calculation. Examine the container and its remaining contents, then the soil on the child's clothing, and the floor where you made the discovery. Make an allowance for the quantity of the spill. Search your memory as to whether this was a partially used container or one which was never previously opened.

QUESTION THE CHILD for the source of the substance if you do not recognize it at all. If you hadn't made him cry, he might lead you to a neighbor's garage or rubbish bin where you might learn about other objects that were also "tasted."

CALL YOUR LOCAL POISON CONTROL CENTER should you have any concern regarding the child's safety. These are information centers especially set up by federal and state agencies to handle problems of this nature. It is well worth the effort to search out that telephone number now. Your local hospital or health department will be glad to give it to you. Then place it in a convenient location with other emergency numbers such as that of your local police and fire departments.

If a local center is not available in your area, the Poison Control Center of the Department of Health of the City of New York is most accommodating. The telephone number is 212–566–8020. Be prepared to give the Poison Control Center the following information in a calm and precise fashion.

1. Age of the child.
2. Approximate weight.
3. Exact and full name of the substance swallowed. It is best to read this from the container label and not trust your memory. The label may also have actual chemical names listed which you can spell out.
4. The size of the container itself; such as four ounces, pint, quart, etc.
5. Your best guess of the amount swallowed.

The Poison Control Center will be able to evaluate the possible danger and advise you accordingly. If medical attention is necessary, they will direct you to the nearest hospital emergency room. By the time you arrive, the personnel at the hospital will have been advised of the nature of the substance swallowed and will be prepared to administer proper care.

Cosmetics pose little or no hazard if swallowed. Creams, lotions or lipsticks, if eaten in large enough quantity (such as one or two tablespoonsful for a twenty-pound child), might cause a few loose bowel movements for a day.

If a child were successful in swallowing enough shampoo to cause him harm, he'd be unable to keep it down—he'd vomit it rapidly.

Perfumes, colognes and toilet waters are alcoholic. If swallowed they would react in the same way as whiskey.

The actual color component of hair coloring products might be hazardous if swallowed in large enough amounts.

Despite the lack of hazard, prevent small children, particularly the toddler, from gaining access to your cosmetics—or any household product not meant for eating.

INDEX

Allergy (*continued*)
    patch test for, 99, 168–171
    photoallergy, 104
    to poison ivy, 98
    to sunlight, 104
Alopecia areata, 17, 214
Aluminum salts, 139–140
Antiperspirants, 139–144
Antiseptics, 61, 244
Astringents, 47, 48, 139
Athlete's foot, *See* Fungus
Atopy, 103–104

Bacteria
    perspiration and, 138, 140–141
    skin and, 56, 138
Baldness, *See* Hair loss
Bathing, 50–53
    See also Skin cleansing
Beard softener, 131
Beer rinse, 161
Benzalkonium chloride, 141
Birthmarks, 72, 148
Blackheads, 41, 54, 55–56, 63–64
Bleaching, *See* Hair coloring
Blemishes, *See* Acne; Blackheads
Blisters, 80, 94, 95, 100, 104, 246
Blood vessels, 28–30
    bathing and, 50, 250
    blushing, 29, 111
    body-heat mechanism and, 79–80
    camouflaging, 111
    capillaries, 28, 84
    dilation by sunburn, 80
    stimulation of, 47–48, 250
Blushers, 125–126
Blushing, 29, 111

Calluses, 32, 246–248
Camomile rinse, 181
Cetalkonium chloride, 141
Chapping, 21, 62, 71
Chemabrasion, 74, 149, 150
Chloasma, 91
Cleansing, *See* Skin cleansing
Cold sores, 102
Colognes, 130, 131, 136, 141
Comedones, *See* Blackheads
Contact dermatitis, 93, 95, 100
Corium, 6, 13, 56
Corns, 32, 246–248
Cortex, hair, 16, 156, 176
Corticosteroids, 158
Cosmetics, 107–133

allergy and, 101–106
application sequence of, 108, 109–129
atopic dermatitis, 103–104
base, 112
blusher, 125–126
eyebrows, 113–115
eyeliner, 118–121·
eyeshadow, 115–118
false eyelashes, 122
foundation, 112–113
hormone products, 71
hypoallergenicity, 101
leg make-up, 250
lipstick, 126–128
making up, 109–129
for males, 129–133
mascara, 122
pregnenalone acetate, 72
removal of, 47, 48, 120, 250
undermake-up moisturizer, 110–111
See also Creams; Hair coloring; Lotions; Skin cleansers; soaps
Creams
antiperspirant, 140
bleaching, 91
bronzer, 89, 132
buffing (nails), 235
cleansing, 44, 244, 250
cuticle remover, 231
deodorant, 141
depilatory, 202
drying, 61
emollient, 71
exotic compound, 72
hair conditioner, 162
medicated, 61
night creams, 44, 49, 71, 72, 132
resorcinol, 61
sulfur, 61
See also Cosmetics; Lotions; Skin cleansers; Soaps

Dandruff, 157
acne and, 64
baldness and, 217
treatment of, 158
Dermabrasion, 74, 149, 150
Deodorants, 130–131, 140–143
Depilatories. *See* Hair removal
Dermis, 6, 13, 29, 68–69
Detergents, 47
in atopic dermatitis, 104
effect on nails, 224
shampoo, 159
synthetic detergent bars, 36–37

Diaper rash, 39
Dihydroxyacetone, 88

Egg rinse, 161
Electrolysis, 204–212
Endocrine system, 54, 56
Environment, effect of
    on aging, 69
    on nails, 224
    on skin, 3, 49
Epidermis, 6, 9–11, 67, 246
Eyes
    circles under, 91–92
    puffiness around, 91
    sun exposure and, 81–82
Eyebrows, 113–115, 209
Eyelashes, *See* False eyelashes
Eyeliner, 118–121
    application of, 118, 125
    removal of, 120
    types of, 118
Eyeshadow, 115–119
    application of, 115
    blending of, 117
    removal of, 120
    types of, 115

False eyelashes, 122–125
    application of, 125
    contouring of, 123
    eyeliner and, 119
    removal of, 125
    types of, 122
Fever sore, 102
Foot care, 242–250
Formaldehyde nail hardeners, 237
Foundations, 112, 113
Freckles, 68, 90, 148
Frostbite, 79
Frosted finish, 115
Fungus, 41–42, 225, 244

Gelatin, 181, 236
Glands
    apocrine (scent), 24–26, 138
    endocrine, 54, 56
    sebaceous (oil), 19, 38–43, 54, 55, 129, 138
    sweat, 22, 38, 39, 40, 43, 138
    thyroid, 139, 225
Growths, *See* Skin growths

Hair, 13–19, 155–122
    beard growth, 54, 195
    brassiness, 178
    breakage, 18, 166, 175, 188, 194, 213

Skin cleansing (*continued*)
of feet and legs, 243–244
for infants, 38–40
soaps and, 35–37
See also Bathing; Soaps
Skin growths
removal of, 72–76
warts, 248–249
Soaps
acne and, 61
aging skin, and, 71
atopic dermatitis, 104
cleansing, 60, 70, 196, 243, 250
deodorant, 141
french (multi-milled), 36
medicated, 37, 61
milled, 35
shampoo, 159
shaving, 197
superfatted, 36
synthetic detergent, 36
transparent, 37
See also Skin cleansing
Static electricity, 161, 163
Steroids, *See* Hormones
Strand test, 172, 186, 192
Stripping, 173–175
See also Hair bleaching and coloring
Sulfur, 61, 158
Sun, 69–70, 77–92
damage caused by, 3, 78, 80–91
dyed hair and, 176
effect on body tissues, 80–85
effect on pigmentation, 81, 90–92
poisoning by, 81
protection of skin from, 85–90
Sun bathing, 70, 87
Sun lamps, 78–79
Sun-protective agents, 70, 86–90
Sweat (ecrine) glands, 22–26, 38, 40, 138, 244
Sweating, *See* Perspiration

Tar, 61, 158
Thioglycolic acid, 185, 203
Thiuram disulfide, 141
Toilet water, 136, 141, 260
Toupee, 217–220
Transplant, hair, 220–222
Turtle oil, 72

Varicose veins, 243
Vitamins, 59, 69

Warts, 248–249

Dr. Earle W. Brauer, noted expert on the relationship between medicine and cosmetology, has been a practicing dermatologist for over twenty years and is currently Medical Director of the Revlon Research Center, Inc., in New York City. He is Associate Professor of Clinical Dermatology at the New York University School of Medicine and Associate Attending Dermatologist at the University Hospital at New York University Medical Center in New York City.